Elizabeth Shaw, MS, RDN
and Chef Sara Haas, RDN, LDN

Fertility
FOODS
COOKBOOK

100+ RECIPES TO NOURISH YOUR BODY

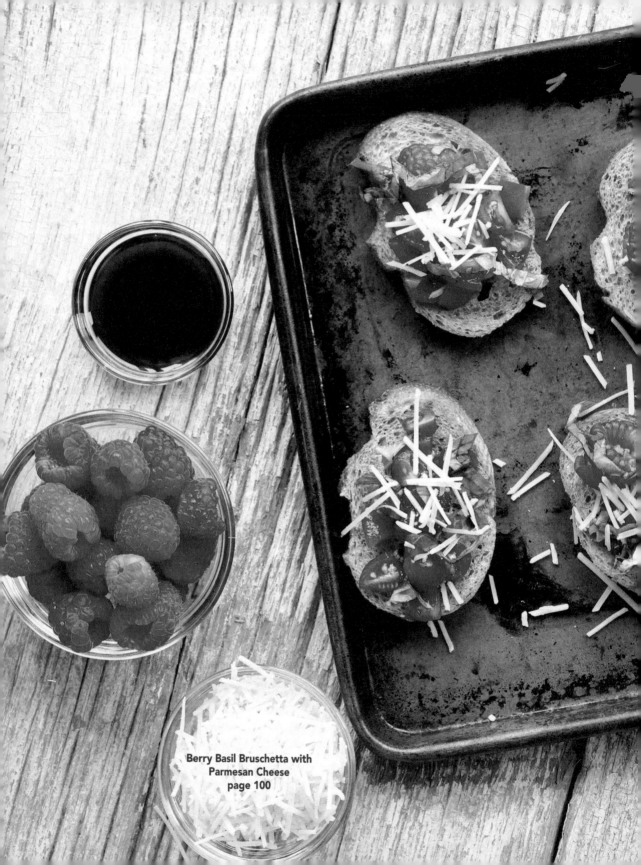

Berry Basil Bruschetta with
Parmesan Cheese
page 100

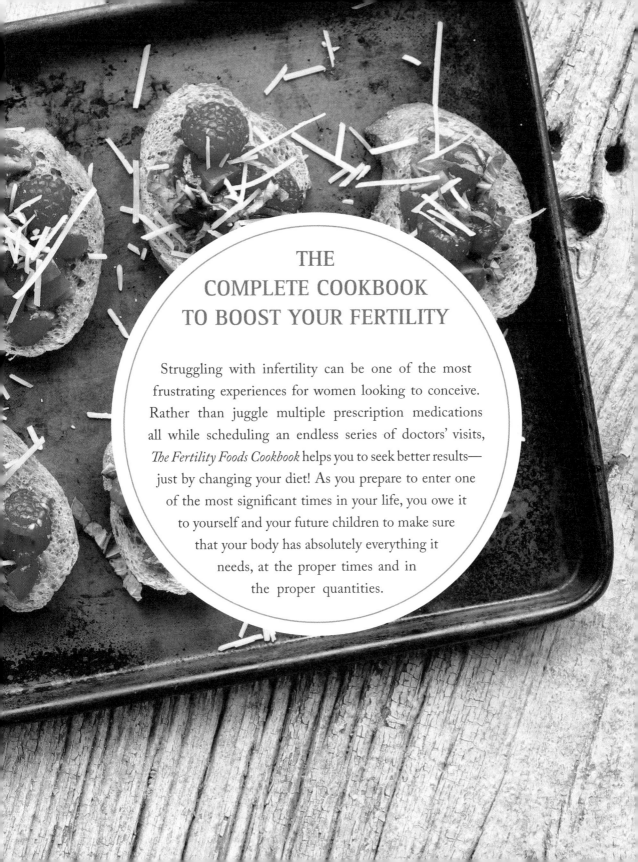

THE
COMPLETE COOKBOOK
TO BOOST YOUR FERTILITY

Struggling with infertility can be one of the most frustrating experiences for women looking to conceive. Rather than juggle multiple prescription medications all while scheduling an endless series of doctors' visits, *The Fertility Foods Cookbook* helps you to seek better results— just by changing your diet! As you prepare to enter one of the most significant times in your life, you owe it to yourself and your future children to make sure that your body has absolutely everything it needs, at the proper times and in the proper quantities.

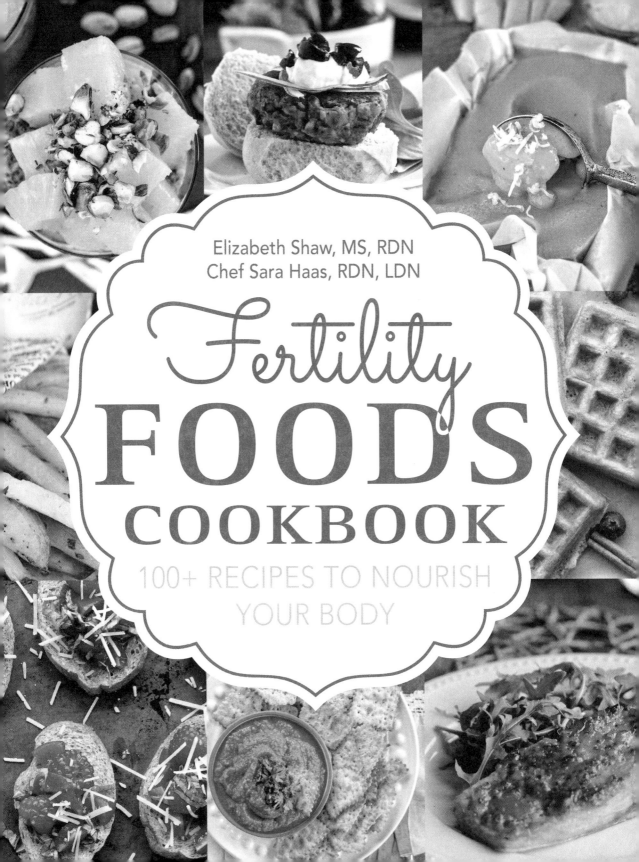

Elizabeth Shaw, MS, RDN
Chef Sara Haas, RDN, LDN

Fertility FOODS COOKBOOK

100+ RECIPES TO NOURISH YOUR BODY

Hatherleigh Press is committed to
preserving and protecting the natural resources of the earth.
Environmentally responsible and sustainable practices are embraced
within the company's mission statement.

Visit us at www.hatherleighpress.com and register online for free
offers, discounts, special events, and more.

FERTILITY FOODS

Library of Congress Cataloging-in-Publication Data is available upon request.
ISBN: 978-1-57826-703-3

COVER AND INTERIOR DESIGN BY CAROLYN KASPER

Printed in the United States
10 9 8 7 6 5 4 3 2

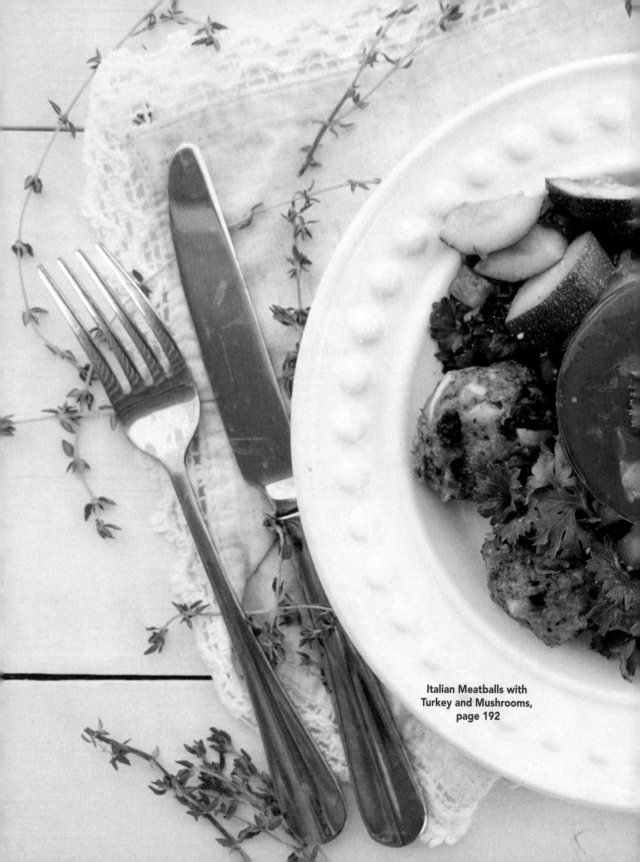

Italian Meatballs with
Turkey and Mushrooms,
page 192

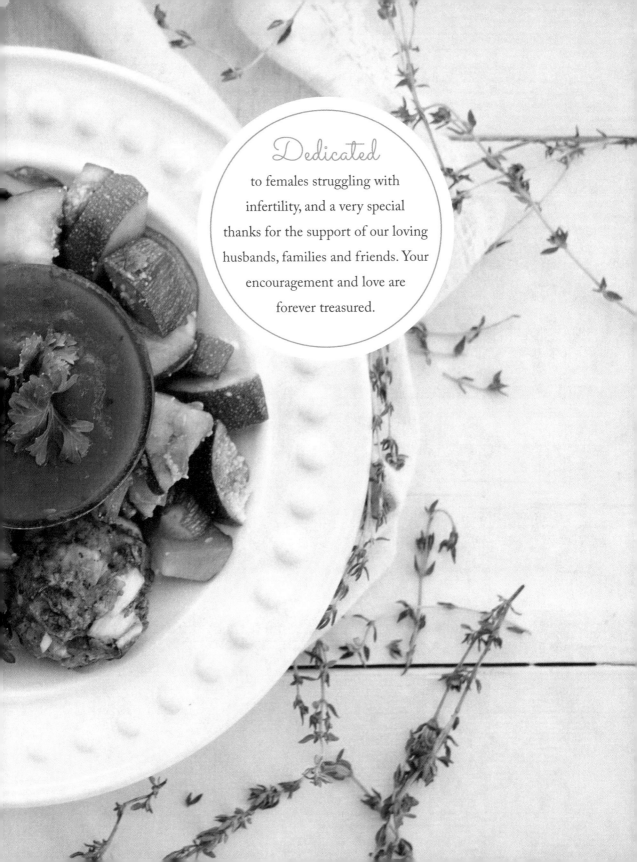

Dedicated

to females struggling with
infertility, and a very special
thanks for the support of our loving
husbands, families and friends. Your
encouragement and love are
forever treasured.

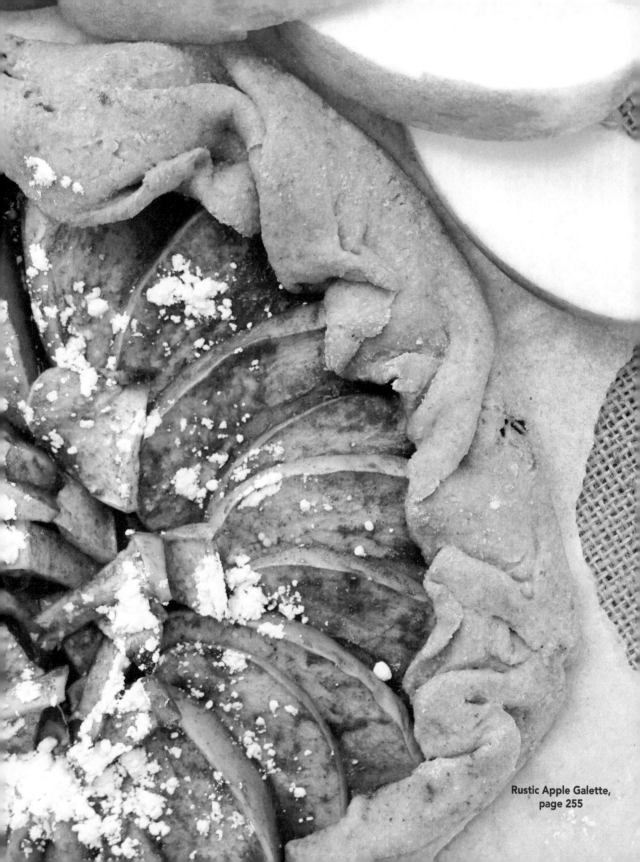

Rustic Apple Galette,
page 255

Contents

Part 1:

THE RECIPE FOR NUTRITION AND FERTILITY

Part 2:

FERTILITY FOOD RECIPES

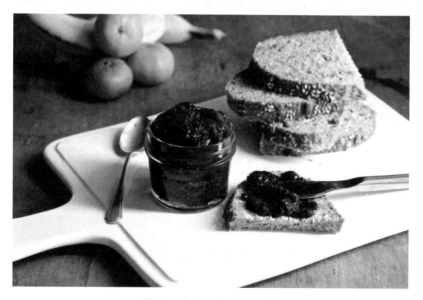

All Natural Berry Jam, page 57

Foreword

I MET THESE TWO REMARKABLE women like many people meet nowadays—on the internet. As fellow health food bloggers, we're part of a large network of people who share a common passion for food and the amazing power that it has to affect our health.

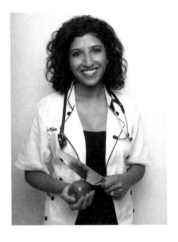

Having treated many pregnant patients in the emergency room over the years, one commonality I've noticed is that women often view pregnancy as the ideal time to make positive changes in their lives. Whether it is quitting smoking, being more physically active, or eating healthier, women have a natural instinct to do what's best for their babies.

When I was researching my book *Natural Pregnancy Cookbook*, I was humbled by the power we have as women to affect not only our own health, but also the health of our developing babies. What I learned from reading *Fertility Foods* is that you can start even earlier. You can prime your body even before conception using the power of food. By no means are the authors guaranteeing pregnancy by reading this book. Rather, they are helping to empower you and teaching you how to fuel your body with the right nutrients so that you are stronger, healthier, and ready when (using their own words) the "bigger plan" comes along.

In this groundbreaking book, the authors set out to explore the relationship between food and fertility. The information and recommendations presented in this book are honest, comprehensive, and backed by science. They break down which important nutrients you need to nourish your body to make sure it's in the optimal condition to fuel your fertility.

And who better to write this book than these two women, with their impressive list of credentials? With their expertise in both the nutrition and culinary worlds, Liz and Sara have both accomplished so much professionally, whether it be through teaching students, consulting, serving as nutrition experts at the national level, or being public personas on the radio and TV. What strikes me the most is their common passion for sharing their knowledge with others. And now they're doing that once again by writing this book and sharing their personal journeys.

The overall sense you get when reading this book is one of friendship and camaraderie, reassuring readers that they've been there, too. They offer helpful advice not only as nutrition experts, but also as women who've gone through fertility struggles themselves.

In addition to the wealth of nutritional information provided, this book also provides valuable tips about basic culinary techniques and food safety, as well as how to stock a healthy kitchen. And finally, it offers a wonderful and diverse collection of nutritious recipes to suit any taste. From breakfast to dinner to sweet treats, there's something for everyone. Whether you're trying the *Carrot Cake Pancakes*, *Umami Burgers* or *Dark Chocolate Cherry Almond "BonBons,"* they'll show you how to create healthy, nourishing meals and have fun doing it. The recipes are easy and approachable and they all include a "fertility focus" detailing why the dish is important to fuel your fertility and give you the energy you need to feel your best.

Infertility can be an unpredictable, bumpy ride with lots of twists and turns. The authors want to take the stress out of an already stressful situation and put the reins in your capable hands. They want to empower you to make smart nutrition choices so that you can nourish yourself properly and prime your body with wholesome, delicious food. So sit back, relax, and take some time to curl up with this book. It will feel like you're catching up with two old friends. And I bet you'll be amazed at how much you learned, too.

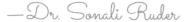

—Dr. Sonali Ruder

Board-certified Emergency Medicine physician, creator of the popular food blog *The Foodie Physician* and author of *Natural Pregnancy Cookbook* and *Natural Baby Food*

Authors' Note

> *"I know God will not give me anything I can't handle. I just wish that He didn't trust me so much."*
>
> — Mother Teresa

D O Y O U E V E R F E E L this way? While you may accept the challenges your life presents, you still have to wonder *why* it has to be so tough, why your burden seems *overly* burdensome.

Don't worry; you're in good company. We all share Mother Teresa's sentiment at times. Early on in our lives, we dealt with our challenges differently; we put in hard work and endless effort, and in doing so, we found success. Perhaps it is no surprise, then, that we found ourselves working so hard at everything. Eventually, we came to equate hard work with success. After all, it seemed applicable in so many areas of our lives. School, sports, friendships—almost everything followed the "rule" that anything is possible if you work hard enough.

So you can imagine our surprise when we found out that this great life skill doesn't apply to infertility.

We firmly believed that if we worked hard enough we would get pregnant. So we worked *really* hard at whatever we thought we could do to improve our odds of getting pregnant. We bought books about infertility; we stopped eating our favorite foods; we changed exercise routines . . . basically, we did everything we could think of to "become more fertile."

And here's what we found: instead of making us feel better, doing all of that made us feel depressed, frustrated, and unhappy. We were putting the maximum effort into becoming the most fertile versions of ourselves (or so we thought)—which was somewhat satisfying in itself—but we'd given up so many of the things that we loved and had nothing to show for it. We found ourselves spending countless hours wondering what we could be doing differently or better.

As you can imagine, that type of behavior is only sustainable for so long. Knowing that we didn't want to head down the path of pity and get trapped in the "why me's", we found other, healthier ways to challenge ourselves and exert our energy. We started blogging about our struggles. We went back to the kitchen to experiment with new recipes. We put faith in Faith, fully believing there was a bigger plan for us. And, finally, we found doctors we loved and trusted.

Infertility and infertility related conditions affect an estimated eighteen percent of all couples who are trying to conceive[1]. That's a staggering statistic, but it at least serves to acknowledge the fact that we're not alone—that *you're* not alone. The path of infertility is challenging and leads to so many unanswerable questions. It's a terrifying and alienating place to be, and you only "get it" if you've gone or are going through it.

TRUST US, WE GET IT!

We get it; we know it's not easy. As fate would have it, our exhausting, terrifying experiences had a silver lining: it afforded us the opportunity to meet, brought together through the blogging world. When we both opened up about our experiences, what we found was an instant connection. We found comfort in sharing our stories with each other and we leaned on one another, and so began a great friendship.

In discussing our respective journeys with each other, we found that we'd both sought to learn more about the relationship between food and fertility, yet neither of us could find anything written by true nutrition professionals, much less anything written by nutrition experts who had gone through the experience of infertility.

It was clear that our mutual passion was to fill that void on the bookstore shelf. We both wanted to help people struggling with infertility realize the power that food can play in their lives. We wanted to write this book to help people like you find a friend in all of this. Through telling our stories, we hope you will realize that you, too, are among friends. That you are not alone.

Yes, we'll say it again. You are not alone! Remember that. We're here to help, and we will constantly remind you of that. Just as we needed to hear those words, we are happy to share them with you. *You are not alone!*

With that said, we're delighted to have you with us, and look forward to sharing this bumpy road together!

Meet Elizabeth Shaw

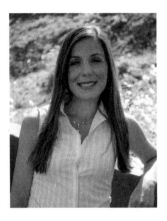

WELCOME! I'M ELIZABETH, BUT please call me Liz. I'm a California native, a registered dietitian nutritionist, and a certified LEAP (Lifestyle Eating and Performance) therapist. I have a Master's degree in dietetics and a graduate certificate in eating disorders and obesity. I work as an adjunct professor of nutrition for the local community college district while also running my own nutrition communications business in San Diego. In this position, I get to have the pleasure of doing a variety of different things, including freelance writing, recipe development, and live broadcasts. I also author two blogs (shawsimpleswaps.com and bumpstobaby.com), though my true passion is the book you now hold in your hands—or, at least, the dream that it represents.

That's my professional background out of the way. But who am I, really?

I am a *healthy* foodie and *wannabe* mamma. I began this book as part of a lifelong goal to tell my story through writing, though I was never quite sure what form that would take. Lo and behold, life happened, and I found myself facing intimidating library shelves, fruitlessly surfing the web, and asking just about every person I knew who'd gone through infertility what I should be reading. Sure, there are plenty of options out there, but nothing that I felt would help me have more control over my situation. At that moment, it became clear to me what form the book inside me would take. I like to think of this as the first part of that bigger plan I mentioned.

Let's rewind a bit so you understand what led me to this point. Early in my life, I was diagnosed with anorexia, having lost over 25 pounds in a two-month period due to the stress of a move. I sought treatment from a great multidisciplinary team that included a registered dietitian nutritionist, a family therapist, and a physician. This group was my rock.

They inspired me to reevaluate my relationship with food and embrace it as nourishment for my body.

However, it wasn't that easy. If you or someone you know has struggled with disordered eating, you already know that there is usually a trigger point that caused the restriction to start, as well as a turning point that inspires a change for the better, switching gears towards recovery. *My* trigger point was when a teenage boy told me, in the *sweetest way possible*, that I was fat and had a pig nose. Tough words to swallow for a twelve-year-old girl on the brink of puberty.

My turning point is none too rosy, either. I remember it so vividly. One night, when my dad had brought home pizza, my mom and I fought over the fact that I had to eat a slice. I can laugh about it now; my husband and I could seriously devour a whole pizza (I recommend the 4-Layer Mexican Pizza on page 204). However, at that point in my life, that single slice felt like poison to me. Tears were shed, harsh words were said, and in a surge of emotion, my mom shouted, "Don't you ever want to have kids, Elizabeth?!"

Those words struck a chord in me like you wouldn't believe. What was she talking about? Of *course* I wanted kids when I grew up. But I was twelve! I was busy focusing on getting my braces off and going to the eighth grade graduation dance.

I realized I needed to change my ways. I began my journey to weight restoration. I knew in my heart that my calling in life was to become a registered dietitian nutritionist, helping others realize the important role nutrition plays in the body.

It's important to point out the key elements of this story—the ones that even now play a critical role in my struggle with infertility. I was just entering puberty when I was diagnosed with anorexia nervosa, meaning my hormones hadn't had the chance to regulate. My physician at the time advised the only way to reconcile my irregular periods was to place me on birth control. Thus, at the tender age of twelve, I began an oral contraceptive regimen that would last for another thirteen years.

This little pill was the Band-Aid that I didn't rip off until I was 24, when I decided that my body could do just fine on its own. I had read it would take a few months for my body to adjust on its own, so I waited. And waited. Then I waited some more. Finally, after nine months, I went to the obstetrician. He ran a few blood tests and an ultrasound to check my uterine lining, and, just as he expected, it was nonexistent!

The only positive in the whole situation was that he *did* see plenty of eggs in my ovaries; they just didn't want to come out. So, after being diagnosed with secondary amenorrhea (the loss of menstruation), he sent me to a reproductive endocrinologist.

I remember the fear I felt deep in my chest. "What is wrong with me?" I fretted. "Why can't I get a period?" I shared these fears with my reproductive endocrinologist, who said I just needed to relax, to let go of the stress in my life. *Find peace*, he counseled. My husband agreed.

Just what a woman wants to hear, right? How could I find peace when the peace I *want* is just to feel like a woman again? Three months later, after a barrage of weekly blood draws, temperature monitoring and weight gain, we found my final diagnosis: hypogonadotropic hypogonadism (HH). Basically, HH is the absence of the female sex hormones that stimulate the menstrual cycle. Without them, you're unable to ovulate. This can be caused by many different situations, likely masked by the aforementioned Band-Aid placed on my menstrual irregularities as a teenager—the pill.

The moral of this story is that the road of life is not without its speed bumps, but you can choose to handle them in many ways. I am choosing to write; to tell my story. To help others find peace, a sense of control, in what can feel like the most out of control situation imaginable.

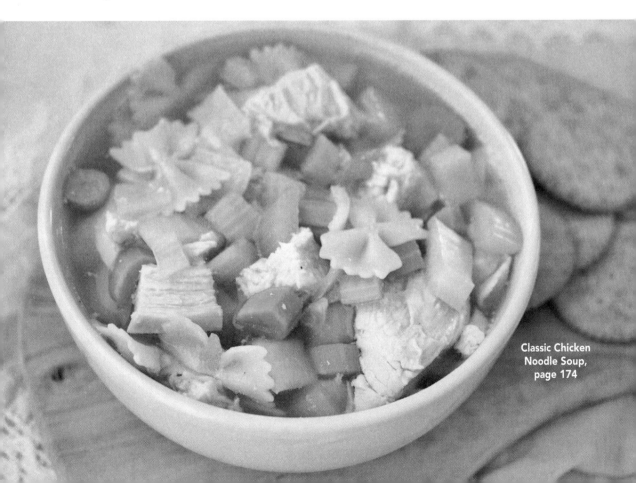

Classic Chicken
Noodle Soup,
page 174

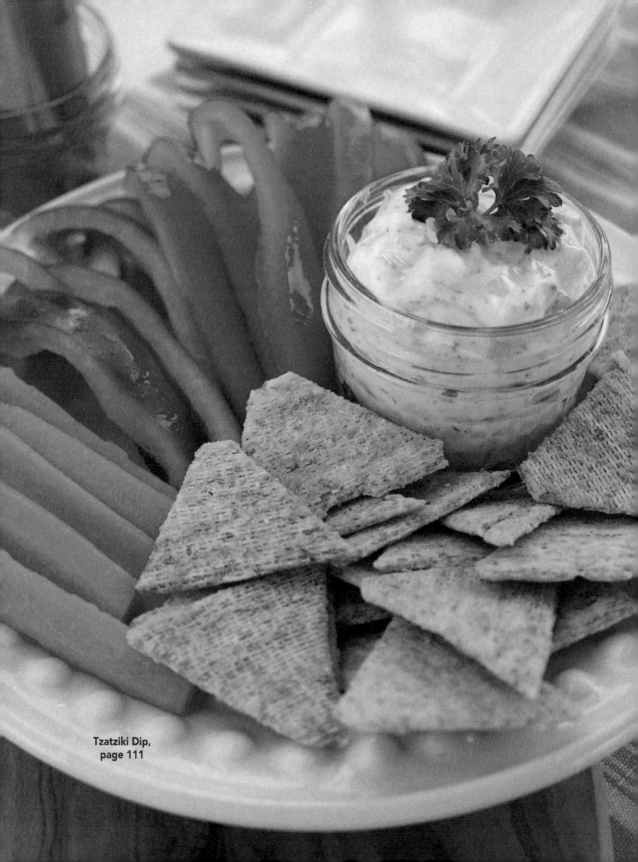

Tzatziki Dip,
page 111

Meet Sara Haas

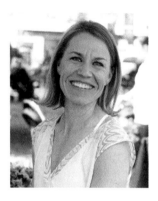

WHY, HELLO THERE! My name is Sara, and I am a registered dietitian nutritionist and classically trained chef living in Chicago, Illinois. My life is a crazy whirlwind, and so is my career. Because of my background, I do a bunch of fun and amazing things, from writing recipes for awesome publications to live cooking demonstrations on television. It certainly keeps me on my toes. I also have a website, sarahaasrdn.com, which features my kitchen creations as well as random thoughts (which are plentiful).

But behind the career, there's a real person, and that's a very special part of who I am.

Here's what I know about my journey through infertility—nothing. I have no idea what caused it or why it happened to me.

Sound familiar?

When I couldn't get pregnant, I kept thinking, "How can this be?" I was perfectly healthy; in fact, my family had always joked that I was the healthiest person they knew. So how could it be that my body, the one that had never failed me, was failing me now? I knew that some people simply have trouble conceiving, but never once did I think that I'd be one of them. It really felt like a slap in the face. I mean, it's our right as women to birth a baby, isn't it?

Let's just say . . . not exactly.

So I don't really know the answer to the eternal question, "Why me?" It could be that a culmination of things, not just one specific element, has contributed to my infertility. But if I had to hazard a guess, it may well have started when I was just a young girl. When I was in the seventh grade, I officially became a woman. Yes, you read that right: at the ripe age of twelve, I went from a kid to a woman—not mentally or emotionally, which might have helped, but physically.

It was downright horrifying. In seventh grade you're supposed to be playing with Barbies and making arts and crafts with your friends, not having to hear "the talk" about how lucky you are to need a bra and wear something called a "pad" in your underwear. I was terrified. I was upset. I hated being different, and I certainly was not ready to be a woman.

Flash forward a few years to high school, when I developed a terrible case of acne. All kids have acne, but mine was devastatingly painful. My face was red, irritated, and blotchy, and I was *beyond* self-conscious about it. Seeing no other solution, my dermatologist recommended starting a drug called Accutane—which *did* work, but Accutane is a serious drug, one that requires frequent blood checks to make sure that everything is okay. It was a quick fix for a nasty problem, but could it have played a role in my infertility? Who can say; but taking extreme prescription drugs for an extended period never seems like a good idea.

Next came the sporadic periods. At the time, I didn't mind that my periods were irregular. Who cared if they came or didn't come? Not me, especially since I'd been "dealing" with them for so long. But towards the end of high school, I visited my nurse practitioner, who thought it would be better if I was more "regular." I didn't ask why, and no diagnosis or testing was done, but at seventeen years old I left with a prescription for "the pill." To "correct the problem," she said. But let's call it what it was: a Band-Aid, one intended for a problem that deserved a diagnosis. Could this be yet another cause for my infertility?

Spring forward about nine years—nine years spent taking oral contraceptives to "keep me regular." I met and married my amazing husband, and stayed on the pill until we decided to start trying to get pregnant. No one had told me to do otherwise, so imagine my surprise when, after going off the pill, I failed to get my period. It was bizarre; I had no idea something like that could happen. After years on the pill, it was as if my body had no idea what it was supposed to be doing on its own.

My obstetrician promptly referred me to a reproductive endocrinologist—an unpleasant and brusque man who, much as my nurse practitioner had done so many years ago, put me on the typical regimen of fertility drugs instead of identifying the cause of my infertility. I should've known better, but I was young and blindly trusted him. Thankfully, my instincts eventually kicked in, and I washed my hands of that practice. They were pushing me towards in-vitro fertilization (IVF), but I wanted to know why I couldn't have a baby naturally.

Luckily, I ended up finding a great reproductive endocrinologist who *did* care about the big WHY, and after ruling out the many probable causes of my infertility, my doctor finally recommended exploratory surgery to see if I had endometriosis (or scar tissue). Of course I agreed; I was scared, but I still wanted those answers, and surgery seemed like the best way to get them.

The results were frustrating. There was indeed some scar tissue—not a lot, but perhaps enough to create a problem—and the "solution" was a drug that would put me into a temporary state of menopause. I was not keen on that, but I wanted a baby, and if endometriosis was in my way, then I wanted to take it out of the equation. I was told to call and order the prescription for the medication, but I delayed doing so. When I did finally call, I learned that it was too late in my cycle to start the medication, and so I would need to wait a month. It was so frustrating; how could I delay this another month?

But fate is a funny thing. That month—the month I was supposed to start the medication that would put me into temporary menopause—was the month I conceived my daughter, naturally, with no medication. A miracle, I thought. And, perhaps, a part of some bigger plan.

I'm on my second journey now, and it's been almost as hard as the first. Just before my daughter's second birthday, we found out we were pregnant. I was so excited but scared at the same time. I made sure to do everything the reproductive endocrinologist advised, but sadly, about two weeks into the pregnancy, I lost my baby. I was devastated. I tried going back to the doctor after that, but all of it was just so *painful*. Visiting that office was just a reminder of my loss. I came to dread waking up early for blood tests, sitting for internal exams and scopes. It depressed me and made me anxious.

We have decided to take the route of a doctorless intervention now in the hopes that, if it is meant to be, it will be. We are focusing on a more holistic approach—revisiting acupuncture, practicing mindfulness and meditation, and spending more time nourishing and nurturing. We vowed to spend more time enjoying the present and the amazing toddler that fills our lives with so much joy. This is the plan for now, to take the pressure off, but we continue praying for another miracle.

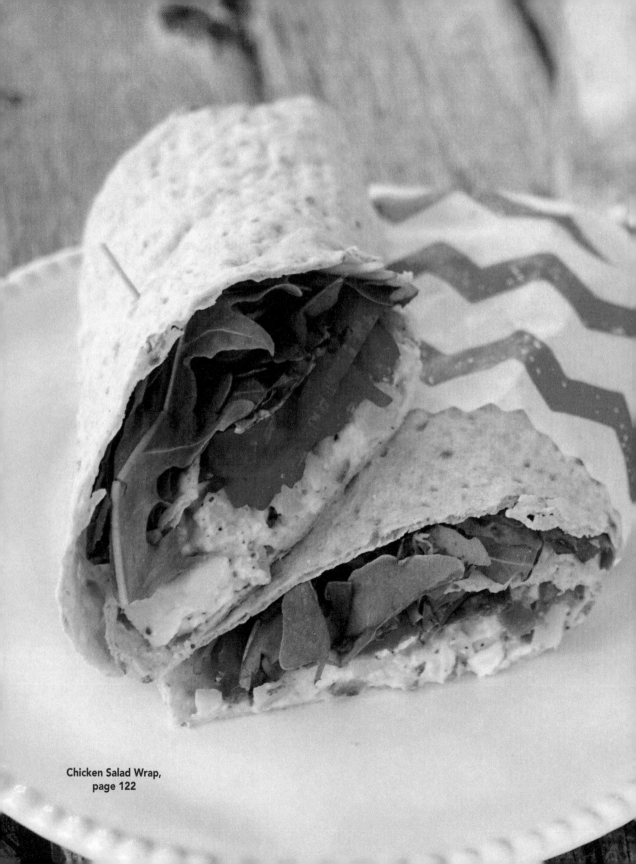

Chicken Salad Wrap,
page 122

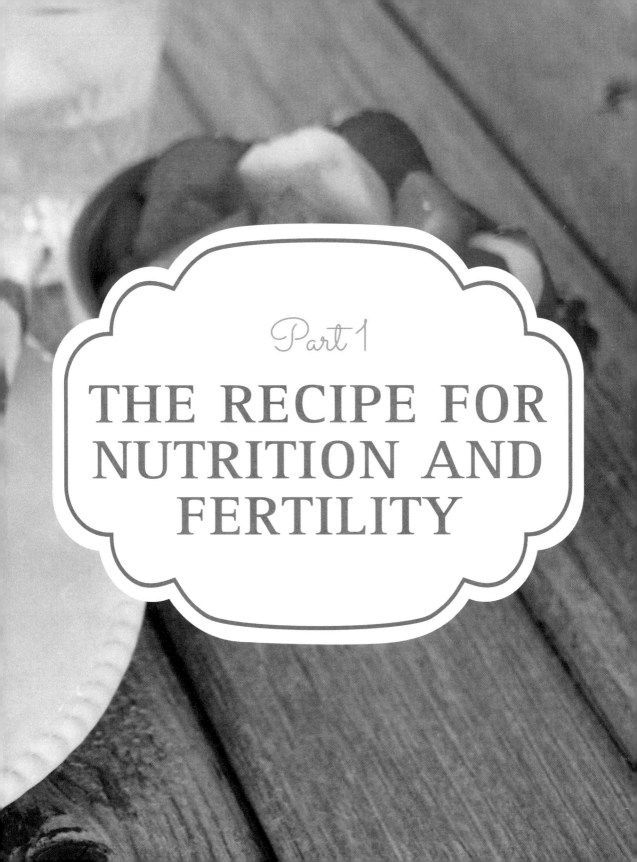

Part 1

THE RECIPE FOR NUTRITION AND FERTILITY

"**H**ELP!"

That's what we yell whenever we fall down, hurt ourselves, feel frustrated, or just need a hand. It's a wonderful word, one that we've used all of our lives, but one that we may have trouble with as we get older. Most of us feel we don't *need* help, that we can handle everything on our own. We've been raised to think that asking for help is a sign of weakness.

But living life like that is hard and stressful. How many times would you have liked help with something but were too stubborn to ask? Help is just what we need when life throws us a curve ball. If you're anything like us, those curve balls make you feel tired, lonely and disheartened. There's only so much you can do on your own before you need help.

That said, help can come in many different forms. Maybe it's a friend who calls to say hello; perhaps it's an article that touches you deeply; it may even be a stranger who holds the door open for you while you're trying to get out of your fifth doctor's visit of the week. The help *we* hope to provide for you in this book is the kind of help we are experts in: nutrition. Better yet, this is the help you can seek in the comfort of your own home.

So sit back, relax, pour yourself a cup of tea, and let us help you.

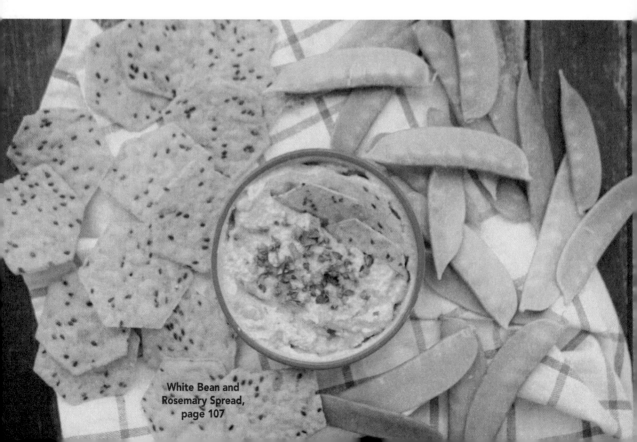

White Bean and Rosemary Spread, page 107

Chapter 1

The Foundation of Food and Fertility

WHAT DO YOU THINK of when you hear the word "nutrition"?

For some, it may spark thoughts of the latest fad diet. For others, it may conjure up memories of their grandma's chicken noodle soup. (You know, the one she used to make that was filled with all those fresh vegetables from her garden? Delicious).

Nutrition is a critical cornerstone of health. Dr. Campbell, author of *The China Study* and the best seller *Whole*, has demonstrated through his research that a void in one nutrient in the body can create a cascade of other nutrient deficiencies and health conditions[2]. As nutrition professionals, we can attest to these findings from what we have seen in our careers.

Yet nutrition remains a controversial topic these days, one that is distorted far too often in the media. It's our goal to provide you with the facts, the backbone of what you need to know at this point in your fertility journey. We're fairly confident this book isn't the first thing you've read about infertility and nutrition. We understand how much information is out there when it comes to this topic. Trust us; we've been there. We've checked out nearly every book in two of the largest cities in the nation (San Diego and Chicago) trying to find *something* relatable—something that breaks down the facts and makes this whole crazy journey seem manageable.

We found a wealth of information that discussed Chinese medicine and Eastern approaches to combat the infertility cycle. It was fascinating how much emphasis is placed on nutrient timing and foods that stimulate blood flow, as well as herbs and tinctures to help infertility. Some books even promise that, in a matter of weeks, you'll find yourself ovulating, practically curing your "infertility" like it never existed.

While the information we read opened our eyes to exploring alternative therapies to treat our conditions, it more often than not left us feeling more confused and out of control. The answers to our nutrition and fertility questions remained vast and unclear.

That's when we decided, once and for all, that nutrition matters! Unless you, too, are a foodie, you may not spend much time thinking about food. Since it's our profession, it's pretty much all we think about. In fact, we were driven to become registered dietitian nutritionists because we believe in the power of food.

THE POWER OF NUTRITION

Think for a moment about how important food truly is. It's more than important, really; it's a necessity. It's what keeps our organs running, our bodies moving, our hearts pumping; it truly gives us life!

Sadly, most of us don't even think twice about the food we eat. But imagine you did start to really consider what you use to fuel the amazing machine that is you. Consider how much control you have over that process, how inspiring it is that you can choose to consume the foods that will make your body perform at its best. It's empowering, isn't it?

It's no lie: what and how you eat impacts your body. We have spent enough hours in clinical nutrition practice, individualized patient care, and behind the scenes in food service to say with confidence that we know the ins and outs of nutrition. That said, as much as we wish we could provide you with a miracle book that could guarantee conception if you read every single page, that's just not realistic, and we don't intend to lie to you.

We *can* promise you, however, that when you do make the nutrition changes we discuss, you will find yourself feeling more in control of your situation. Your body will be ready and willing to accept conception, should the bigger plan roll that way.

NUTRITION AND THE MIND-BODY CONNECTION

Let's take a step back and examine the idea of the whole mind-body connection—that the state of your body affects your mind, and vice versa. It's amazing to think that one of the most important factors that physicians correlate with infertility is stress.

Amazing, but perhaps not so surprising; what isn't stressful these days! We're stressed because we're running late; the dog didn't get a walk; the pizza man didn't deliver in 30 minutes; your co-worker threw you under the bus, again. Stressful situations are going to arise whether we like it or not; that's out of our control. However, how we *manage* that stress is something we can control. That's where nutrition and lifestyle factors come into play.

Has your doctor ever said, "Go ahead and eat all the potato chips and soda you want?" Probably not. (At least, we hope not!) In order to keep your body working at its best, you have to give it the proper nutrients it needs to function. It's no different from a high-class automobile: if you fill it with the wrong kind of fuel, it's going to clank and clatter until it breaks. That doesn't sound like a nice environment for a baby to grow, does it? We don't think so either.

The first step in the process is to make sure *you* are well nourished. When you're at your nutritional best, you will start to feel better and other parts of your life will seem better. Perhaps eating the right food will boost your mood or lead you to a state of relaxation. Food is a powerful part of this process! Recognizing the role that your emotions play in your relationship with food will help make this process a whole lot easier in the long run.

NUTRITION PREP COURSE FOR FERTILITY

We'd love to be there with you every day, cooking with you to make you the healthiest you can be, but as that's just not possible, we hope you'll settle for everything we've put into the making of this book. In the next two chapters, we'll give you the fundamental information you need to help make you the best momma-to-be you can be, guiding you to feel POWERFUL when making your daily food choices.

We want to arm you with nutrition knowledge that will allow you to "own" your own health! We'll teach you about fertility foods and why they're an important part of your health. And we've also put together over a hundred recipes and a collection of resources to let you put this information into action! Our hope is that once you try these for yourself, you'll be able to take what you've learned and create your own inspiring dishes. We want you to see *the big picture* when it comes to being your most well-nourished self. We told you, you're not alone!

Nourishing your body is one thing you can control in this often-unpredictable roller coaster ride of infertility. Regardless of how crazy things feel, taking time to provide your body with wholesome, delicious, and nutritious foods is one of the best ways to regain that sense of calm and control and provide yourself with the strength you need to keep pursuing your baby dreams.

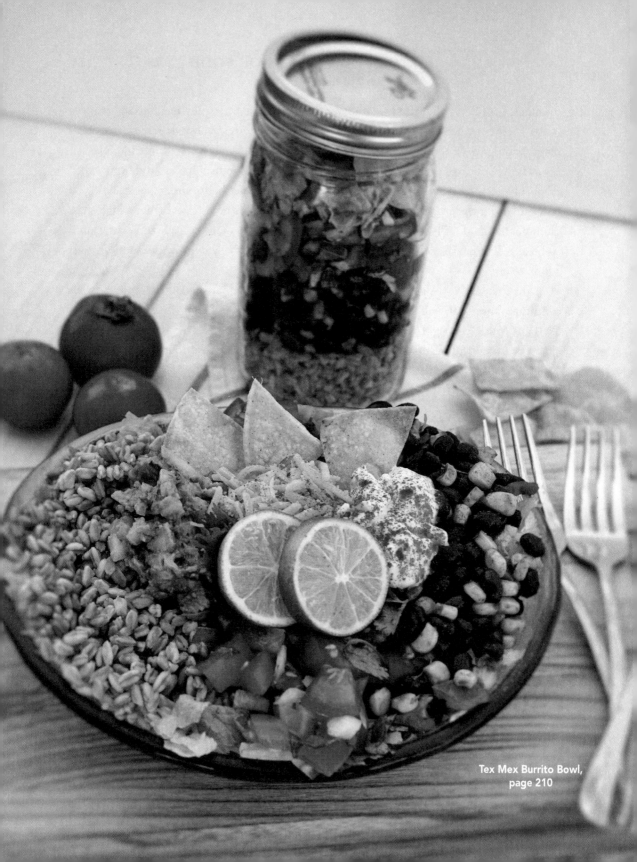

Tex Mex Burrito Bowl,
page 210

Chapter 2

The Main Ingredients

THE EVOLUTION OF MYPLATE

Remember the old food guide pyramid? You know, the little triangle shaped icon from 1992 that helped guide us to eating more healthfully. It showed us that the bulk of our diets, illustrated in the bottom and biggest tier, should consist of grains, followed by the tier of fruits and vegetables, then dairy and proteins and, at the very top, fats and sugars. The dwindling size of the tiers as they approached the top represented the decreased need for that particular food group.

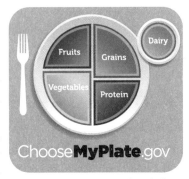

Source: U.S. Department of Agriculture

As nutrition science improved, it was necessary to update the pyramid to reflect new research. Though the original principles (eating fruits and vegetables, whole grains, and healthy fats) were still applicable, the pyramid needed a facelift—which it received in 2005, when it got turned on its side. Exercise was finally included, which further improved the program, but things still weren't quite right.

It was at this point that the United States Department of Agriculture decided to do away with pyramids entirely with the most recent upgrade. Enter MyPlate[4].

Have you heard of MyPlate? If you haven't, that's okay; that's what we're here for! MyPlate is a helpful resource, one that we trust and something we know will help you.

Look at the figure above. Don't you already feel less overwhelmed than when you were looking at that pyramid? A team of scientists and health researchers decided that a plate is the perfect way to communicate how people should be eating. After all, people eat food on a plate, so why not educate them using a tool they are already familiar with? It's genius, really.

Here's the deal: in general, MyPlate instructs that you fill fifty percent of your plate with fruits and vegetables, twenty-five percent of your plate with lean proteins, and the remaining twenty-five percent with whole grains. Outside the plate, you'll notice there's a spot for dairy, too. See? Easy!

Incorporating MyPlate into your diet is an important piece of fueling your fertility because when you practice eating a variety of foods from all groups, you will not only feel better, have more energy, and stress less, but you'll also be more at peace, letting you accept those bigger plans should they come knocking at your door.

Plus, these guidelines are applicable to everyone in your family! A study published in 2012 in *Human Reproduction* found that diets rich in whole grains, fruits, vegetables, chicken, and fish is an inexpensive way to improve semen quality, demonstrating the powerful effect a balanced diet can play in male infertility, too[5]. This means you won't need to spend countless hours in the kitchen making one meal for yourself and another for your loved one(s). Excellent, right?

FRUITS AND VEGETABLES

It's no surprise that of all the MyPlate food groups, Fruits and Vegetables is one of our favorites. Don't worry if you're not a huge fan of fruits and vegetables right now; we promise, by the end of the recipe collection you will be!

There is good reason that fifty percent of the MyPlate graphic consists of fruits and vegetables (or, as we like to call them, the produce patch!). Fruits and vegetables are natural vitamin and mineral powerhouses that, when eaten regularly, can improve your overall health and wellness. Countless research studies conducted over the years have proven time and time again that eating more fruits and vegetables will make you a healthier human being; that's something we all long for, right?

But there *is* some confusion surrounding our produce patch that stems from misinformation in the media. Mixed messages have led many to believe that fruit contains too much sugar and that organic produce is the "only way to go." It's disheartening for us as registered dietitians to hear *any* fresh fruit or vegetable labeled "bad" or considered "off limits." The bottom line: we all need to eat more fruits and vegetables, and a variety of them, too! Here's a quick glance at the types of fruits and vegetables (and their sources) that health professionals refer to as members of the produce patch.

FRUITS & VEGETABLES

- Fresh
- Canned
- Frozen
- Dried
- Pureed
- 100% Juice

You see? Fruits and vegetables can be enjoyed in so many ways. Fresh is great, but you should also feel good about consuming fruits and vegetables in their canned, frozen, dried, and juice forms. That said, you *will* need to pay attention to labels and ingredient lists, and choose varieties with no added sugar, which can be variously labeled as "high fructose syrup," "cane juice," "brown rice syrup," and "dextrose." As for canned or frozen vegetables, sodium can often be a concern, so read labels to be sure you're purchasing "low sodium" or "no salt added" varieties.

In addition, when it comes to vegetables, not all are created equal—there are some that are considered "starchy" vegetables, including potatoes, winter squash, and corn. Although most vegetables contain small amounts of carbohydrates in their chemical makeup, these starchy vegetables contain higher amounts. This is especially important when it comes to anyone with pre-diabetes or diabetes: unlike other vegetables, starchy vegetables contain more carbohydrates that will cause a rise in blood sugar.

CHOOSING FRUITS AND VEGETABLES FOR FERTILITY

ORGANIC VS. CONVENTIONAL

It's important we take a minute and discuss a hot topic in nutrition today: organic vs. conventional foods. As registered dietitian nutritionists, our job is to remind you that fruits and vegetables are a great source of nourishment and that consuming them should remain a top priority in order to optimize your health.

Now, should you purchase organic? The answer is yes . . . and no. (Gosh, we really couldn't make it easy for you, could we? Sorry, friends, it's just not that black and white.) Recently published research suggests decreased sperm quality owing to higher intakes of pesticide residue-containing produce[6]. However, the study also showed that men who ate low to moderate pesticide containing produce had a higher number of morphologically normal sperm. Studies such as this make it hard to issue a blanket statement regarding whether or not you should always purchase organic.

If you want to err on the side of caution while going through this roller coaster of infertility, we suggest taking a look at the Environmental Working Group (EWG), a nonprofit organization devoted to arming the public with knowledge and research regarding issues of public health and environmental concerns[7]. Each year an updated list is published that evaluates the levels of pesticides found in various fruits and vegetables. The results are then categorized into two lists: the "Clean 15" and "Dirty Dozen." Here's a look at the most recent findings:

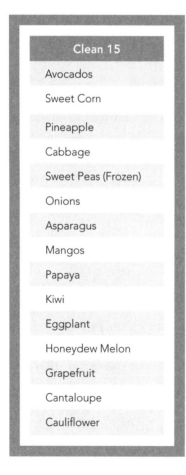

Clean 15
Avocados
Sweet Corn
Pineapple
Cabbage
Sweet Peas (Frozen)
Onions
Asparagus
Mangos
Papaya
Kiwi
Eggplant
Honeydew Melon
Grapefruit
Cantaloupe
Cauliflower

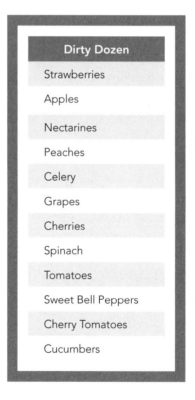

Dirty Dozen
Strawberries
Apples
Nectarines
Peaches
Celery
Grapes
Cherries
Spinach
Tomatoes
Sweet Bell Peppers
Cherry Tomatoes
Cucumbers

Both organic and conventional produce are nutrient dense and necessary in a balanced diet to achieve optimum health. That said, what do we do in *our* homes?

Liz: Personally, I do not always purchase organic when it comes to the Dirty Dozen. It can get expensive and, to be honest, the literature is not conclusive enough to show a direct correlation in conventional produce and infertility rates. Findings from alternative studies, such as the 2011 Journal of Toxicology, showed that twenty-three percent of organic food samples also tested positive for pesticide residue[8]. Thus, I buy organic when I can, but it's not always a priority for me.

Sara: When it comes to the Dirty Dozen, I choose to purchase organic. Research is ongoing regarding pesticides and their link to infertility and, since findings of the effect of pesticides on the reproductive system are concerning, I prefer to proceed with caution and fill my refrigerator with the organic varieties.

The question comes down to personal choice, and we encourage you to be an informed consumer. Do your due diligence in terms of research so that you can make informed decisions that make sense for you and your family.

THE BIGGER PICTURE OF PRODUCE

What *is* conclusive are the studies that show a positive correlation with a healthy, balanced diet—one high in fruits and vegetables—and benefits on fertility[9]. The plethora of colors found in plant foods actually contain many important nutrients, also known as "phyto (or plant) nutrients." It's amazing to think that plants naturally contain over 4,000 phytonutrients (which include antioxidants), all with specific benefits for our body[10]. Produce like tomatoes, leafy greens, and mushrooms naturally contain antioxidants that help fight free radicals, the "bad guys" that can damage our body's healthy cells.

Free radicals are created as a result from our exposure to UV light, air pollution and smoke. But it's not just the environment we have to blame: free radicals are also formed as a natural byproduct of your body's metabolism. These unstable molecules wreak havoc, searching and stealing charged particles from healthy cells and weakening their structure and function. Over time, this constant barrage to healthy cells can cause serious damage, leading to the development of chronic disease (such as cancer), and can place your body in a state of oxidative stress.

Infertility is often seen in individuals with high levels of oxidative stress. For this reason, a high intake of antioxidant-containing fruits and vegetables may benefit your fertility[11].

What does this mean for you? It means that there's no time better than now for you to start "eating the rainbow!" The handy chart below showcases the variety of health benefits you'll enjoy by consuming an array of the phytonutrients that come from these amazing fruits and vegetables[12]. Refer to it before your next trip to the grocery store.

Color	Food	Phytonutrient	Importance
Blue/Purple	Eggplant, blueberries, blackberries, prunes, plums, pomegranates, purple cabbage	Anthocyanins	Antioxidant, promotes heart health, supports healthy blood pressure and may help prevent clot formation
Green	Broccoli, green cabbage, bok choy, Brussels sprouts	Isothiocyanates	Antioxidant, helps rid the body of potentially carcinogenic compounds
Yellow/Green	Avocado, kiwifruit, spinach and other leafy greens, pistachios	Lutein	Antioxidant, promotes eye and heart health, protects against cancer
Red	Tomatoes and tomato products, cranberries, watermelon, pink grapefruit	Lycopene	Antioxidant, reduces risk of some cancers and has cardio-protective properties
Yellow/Orange	Carrots, mangos, winter squash, sweet potatoes, pumpkins, apricots	Beta-cryptoxanthin, beta carotene, alpha carotene (carotenoids)and vitamin C	Antioxidant, anti-inflammatory properties, essential for conversion of vitamin A to promote eye health
Colorless	Berries, grapes, spinach, onions, apples, celery, bell peppers, Brussels sprouts, citrus fruits, tea, red wine, dark chocolate	Flavonoids	Rich in antioxidant, rids the body of free radical damage that can inhibit fertility

PORTION SIZES AND RECIPE RECOMMENDATIONS

Now that you know the important role fruits and vegetables play in your fertility, we want to show you how easy it is to design produce-packed meals using the recipes in this book. The table below provides information on serving sizes and can direct you to recipes using a particular fruit or vegetable. Helpful and practical, right? Keep a special lookout for the fruits and vegetables tagged with a (*) below; this means they are a great source of antioxidants!

FRUITS	Amount Equivalent to 1 Cup	Amount Equivalent to ½ Cup	Recipe Recommendation
Whole Fruit (Apple, Peach, Pear, Nectarine)*	1 small/ medium (2¼ inch diameter)	½ cup sliced, raw, chopped, cooked (applesauce)	Lacinato Kale Salad with Peaches and Maple Vinaigrette (page 154)
Berries*	1 cup (8 strawberries)	½ cup berries	Strawberry Banana Smoothie (page 140)
Bananas	1 large (7–9 inches long)	1 small (<6 inches long)	Banana Mango Sorbet (page 247)
Grapes	1 cup (32 seedless)	½ cup (15 seedless)	Freeze as a snack
Melons, Pineapple	1 cup balls, slices	½ cup balls, slices	Pair with Protein Packed Freezer Burritos (page 212) for a quick meal!
100% Fruit Juice*	1 cup	½ cup	All Natural Berry Jam (page 57)
Dried Fruit	½ cup	¼ cup (1½ ounces)	Homemade Granola Bars (page 136)

* = contains antioxidants

VEGETABLES	Amount Equivalent to 1 Cup	Amount Equivalent to ½ Cup	Recipe Recommendation
Broccoli*	1 cup raw or cooked, 3 large spears	½ cup	Broccoli Cheese Soup (page 173)
Brussels sprouts*	1 cup raw or cooked	½ cup	Roasted Vegetables (page 223)
Cauliflower*	1 cup raw or cooked	½ cup	Open Faced Cauliflower Grilled Cheese (page 120)
Carrots*	1 cup strips, 2 medium carrots, 12 baby carrots	1 medium carrot, 6 baby carrots	Carrot Cake Pancakes (page 90)
Corn**	1 cup, 1 large ear (8–9 inches long)	½ cup	Black Bean Salad with Honey-Lime Vinaigrette (page 152)
Cucumbers	1 cup raw or sliced	½ cup raw or sliced	Indian Cucumber Salad with Creamy Yogurt Dressing (page 149)
Leafy Greens* (Spinach, Kale)	1 cup cooked, 2 cups raw	½ cup cooked, 1 cup raw	French Lentil Salad with Spinach and Feta (page 158)
Tomatoes*	1 large raw tomato (3 inch diameter), 1 cup chopped or sliced, raw, cooked or canned	1 small raw tomato (<2 inch diameter), ½ cup chopped or sliced, raw, cooked or canned	Pico de Gallo Salsa (page 114)
Sweet Potatoes	1 large (2¼ inch diameter), 1 cup cooked	½ large (2¼ inch diameter) ½ cup cooked	Sweet Potato Pie Parfait (page 257)
White Potatoes**	1 large (3¼ inch diameter), 1 cup cooked	½ large (3¼ inch diameter), ½ cup cooked	Oven Baked French Fries (page 228)

*= contains antioxidants; ** = considered a "starchy" carbohydrate

GRAINS

Oh, grains, how we love thee! Maybe it's Liz's Italian roots or Sara's German genes, but it turns out this is one of our favorite food groups. And it's a good thing, too: grains are a big group, one that encompasses so many great foods.

But we're getting ahead of ourselves. What *are* grains?

Grains are foods made from wheat, rice, oats, barley, cornmeal and/or other cereal grains. There are two types of grains—whole grains and refined grains (including enriched and fortified)—and it's important for you to know the difference between them.

WHOLE GRAINS

If you're in search of a grain that has it all, look no further than whole grains. Whole grains haven't been milled like refined grains, meaning that the grain is fully intact. Because the grain is whole and intact, that means it contains all three parts of the kernel: the bran, the germ and the endosperm. That's a huge nutritional bonus!

Take a look below and see what we mean!

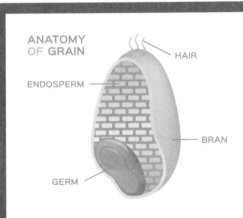

ANATOMY OF GRAIN

HAIR

ENDOSPERM

BRAN

GERM

The Bran: The outer "shell" of the whole grain. Serves to protect the grain against weather, insects, and disease.

Contains: B Vitamins, fiber, copper, magnesium, zinc, iron and antioxidants

The Germ: Where the embryo of the whole grain kernel lives. If fertilized, it will sprout and become a plant.

Contains: protein, healthy fats, Vitamin E, minerals and B Vitamins

The Endosperm: Found just below the surface of the bran, this is the largest part of the kernel and acts as an energy source for the growing plant.

Contains: mostly carbohydrates, protein and some vitamins and minerals

NUTRIENTS FOUND IN WHOLE GRAINS AND THEIR FUNCTIONS

- **B Vitamins:** Metabolism (energy production); maintenance of healthy tissues and organs; red blood cell production (red blood cells supply oxygen to your cells). Includes Thiamin, Niacin, Riboflavin, Vitamin B6 and B12.

- **Fiber (soluble and insoluble):** Important for digestive health; helps prevent constipation; boosts satiety; supports heart health; helps control blood sugar.

- **Vitamin E:** Antioxidant functions that help build your immune system and fend off free radicals.

- **Magnesium:** Helps with nerve impulses, body temperature regulation, detoxification, immunity, energy production, and the formation of healthy bones and teeth.

- **Iron:** Provides oxygen to our cells to facilitate growth and life.

- **Zinc:** Enhances immunity, skin health, as well as maintaining the sensory organs (taste and smell).

- **Copper:** Important for antioxidants in the body, bone and tissue integrity, energy support and cholesterol balance.

REFINED GRAINS

Congratulations, you're a whole grains expert! Now it's time to learn the difference between a whole grain and a *refined* grain.

As we mentioned above, grains are made up of three parts—the bran, the germ and the endosperm. When grains are milled, the bran and germ are removed, and only the carbohydrate-rich endosperm remains. At this point, it's no longer a "whole grain" and is now referred to as a refined grain product. The process creates a fine-textured flour, one that has more stability in terms of shelf life. But to gain that fine texture, you lose out on those important nutrients we discussed.

Refined grains lack nutrient density (in other words, they don't have a lot of bang for their buck, nutritionally speaking). Research suggests that refined grain consumption should be limited for women struggling with infertility[13, 14]. Though we certainly aren't saying you can't have your favorite bagel and cream cheese on occasion, we recommend making mostly nutrient-dense food choices that will provide you with the best fuel for optimum fertility.

Here's a look at some common sources of refined grains.

REFINED GRAIN SOURCES

- Bread, Bagel, Pita: white, wheat, honey wheat, sourdough, Italian (notice we didn't say "whole wheat here!)
- Biscuits
- Crackers
- Ready-to-Eat Cereals (cereals where whole grains/flours are not listed as ingredients)
- Granola Bars
- Cookies, Pastries

ENRICHED AND FORTIFIED GRAINS

When the nutrients removed from grains through the milling process (folic acid, niacin, riboflavin, thiamin and iron) are added back to the grain post-processing, they become "enriched grains." Because of the refining process, enriching foods became necessary, as the removal of these important nutrients led to nutritional deficiencies. While enriching food is beneficial, it doesn't necessarily result in a grain that is as nutritious as a whole grain; one reason being that fiber is not added back after processing. Besides enriching grains, some manufacturers choose to fortify, or add extra nutrients, making the new product a "fortified grain."

Fortification isn't done to grains alone; it occurs with some plant-based milks and fruit juices, too, such as orange juice.

The table below illustrates where these types of grains fall in terms of nutrition.

	Whole Grains	Refined Grains	Enriched Grains	Fortified Grains
Bran	X			
Germ	X			
Endosperm	X	X	X	X
Fiber	X			X
B vitamins (thiamin, riboflavin, niacin, folic acid)	X		X	X
Iron	X		X	X
Added vitamins, minerals				X

CHOOSING THE RIGHT GRAIN FOR FERTILITY

The Dietary Guidelines for Americans recommend at least fifty percent of your daily grains should be whole grains. However, as registered dietitian nutritionists, we know you can do better—and we're prepared to explain how! We recommend you aim for at least seventy-five percent of your grains to be whole grains. Eating more whole grains will not only leave you feeling more satiated (full) after eating, but will also provide a variety of essential vitamins, minerals and other nutrients needed to conceive and foster a healthy pregnancy. Research indicates that diets high in whole grains can improve your fertility[13,14]. For those who are considering IVF, there are further studies that demonstrate a higher intake of whole grains prior to treatment results in a higher probability of live births[15].

Another benefit of eating whole grains is the effect they have on blood sugar. Whole grains do not cause as drastic of a rise in blood sugar as their refined counterparts. Why? Because their chemical structure is more complex than refined grains, meaning it takes your body longer to digest them. Chronic consumption of highly refined carbohydrates (including high sugar foods) over time can lead to insulin resistance and eventually diabetes.

Whole grains have the potential to help with male infertility, as well. Recent research surrounding sperm concentration, motility, morphology, and overall quality suggests that men who choose to follow a diet high in whole grains, as well as fruits, vegetables, legumes and lean proteins (like chicken and fish), have higher sperm quality[5]. As we mentioned, we examined countless books and studies of foods recommended in both Eastern and Western medicine to help facilitate fertility. From that, we found that in the Asian culture, grains are considered the center of the food plate. Whole grains support finding the "golden mean," a place of receptivity, relaxation and mental focus[16]. What a wonderful thought, right? It should therefore come as no surprise that we use so many whole grains in our recipes!

As a special note: individuals with celiac disease or gluten intolerance may have a higher risk of infertility related to their condition[17]. For individuals with such concerns, we recommend speaking with a registered dietitian nutritionist and your physician so they can provide proper support for you and your specific needs.

PORTION SIZES AND RECIPE RECOMMENDATIONS

According to the USDA MyPlate guidelines, a one-ounce serving of grain is considered one portion[3]. Depending on your age, activity level, and individual dietary needs, the recommended number of servings to consume each day will vary. (We'll chat about this more in Part 2, don't worry!) You should also know that there is an amazing variety of whole grain foods available today. In fact, foods that haven't been popular in centuries or that have been virtually unknown to us are resurfacing and can now easily be found in many large chain grocery stores. We encourage you to try these ancient, nourishing grains, such as quinoa, amaranth, and kamut (refer to page 224 for a greater look at other whole grains). Not only are they budget-friendly, but they provide powerful sources of nutrition to help you achieve your most fertile self.

Below is a general guide on portion sizes for whole grain foods. To inspire you to increase your consumption of whole grains, we've included recipes for you to try as you aim to make seventy-five percent of your daily grains whole grains.

WHOLE GRAIN FOODS	Amount Equivalent to 1 Ounce	Common Portions and Ounce Equivalents	Recipe Recommendation
Whole Grain Bread	1 slice	2 slices = 2 ounces	*Fast Veggie and Hummus Sandwich (page 117)*
Whole Grain English Muffin	½ muffin	1 muffin = 2 ounces	*Spinach, Mushroom and Goat Cheese Frittata (page 73)*
100% Whole Grain Products	Approximately 6 crackers	1 handful = 2 ounces	*Garlic Hummus (page 103)*
100% Whole Grain/Wheat Flour	¼ cup	1 small donut, cookie = 2 ounces	*Toasted Coconut Waffles (page 94)*
Brown Rice	½ cup cooked, 1 ounce dry	1 cup cooked = 2 ounces	*Tex Mex Burrito Bowl (page 210)*
Couscous	½ cup cooked	1 cup cooked = 2 ounces	*Grecian Grain Bowl (page 208)*
Whole Grain Muffin	1 small (2½ inch diameter)	1 medium (3½ inch diameter) = 3 ounces	*Chocolate Chip Banana Bread (or muffins) (page 84)*
Whole Grain Pancakes	1 pancake (4½ inch diameter)	2 pancakes = 2 ounces	*Light and Fluffy Whole Wheat Pancakes (page 89)*
Whole Grain Pasta	½ cup cooked, 1 ounce dry	1 cup cooked = 2 ounces	*Parmesan Pesto Pasta with Cherry Tomatoes (page 183)*
Popcorn	3 cups popped, 2 tablespoons kernels	6 cups popped = 2 ounces	*Snack Ideas (page 98)*

WHOLE GRAIN FOODS	Amount Equivalent to 1 Ounce	Common Portions and Ounce Equivalents	Recipe Recommendation
Rolled Oats	½ cup cooked, ⅓ cup dry oats	1 cup cooked = 3 ounces	Homemade Granola Bar (page 136)
Quinoa	½ cup cooked, ¼ cup dry	1 cup cooked = 2 ounces	Mediterranean Veggie Burger (page 124)
Whole Grain Waffles	1 waffle (4½ inch diameter)	2 waffles = 2 ounces	Whole Wheat Freezer Waffles (page 92)
Wild Rice	½ cup cooked, 1 ounce dry	1 cup cooked = 2 ounces	Turmeric Wild Rice Pilaf (page 238)

Though we mentioned refined grains are not as nutritious as their whole grain counterparts, they *do* serve a purpose in certain situations. For instance, if you feel nauseous or light-headed and need a quick release energy source, a refined grain option would be a suitable choice. But how can we say that, after we just got through saying that refined grains were "no good," nutritionally speaking? Well, this is a unique situation: the composition of a slice of white bread or a handful of plain crackers is ideal because they contain minimal fiber, protein and fat. This makes it easier for your body to digest when your body is in a physical state of distress. Hence, the recommendation for eating these foods helps provide calories (energy) while minimizing the stress placed on your digestive system.

DAIRY

We're fairly certain you've already heard your fair share about this food group. Don't worry, we're here to bring you the facts and help you to sort through what you need to know at this stage of your fertility journey.

First things first: what counts as dairy? The dairy group includes milk, yogurt, cheese, ice cream, and calcium-fortified soymilk alternatives. The MyPlate recommendations continue to encourage adults to consume at least three servings of low-fat dairy foods per day, though there is current research that indicates this might not be the case for every individual[18].

What we *do* know is that, when it comes to fertility, dairy (specifically milk) can play a very important role. While dairy is not as large as the other food groups, its size is no indication of its importance.

Here's a look at the important nutrients dairy contains and the roles they play in our body[19,20]:

NUTRIENT	ROLE
Calcium	Growth and maintenance of bones and teeth, nerve functioning, blood clotting
Vitamin D	Supports calcium and phosphorus in promoting bone health
Phosphorus	Supports healthy bones and teeth, key role in cells' genetic material and energy transfer
Riboflavin	Helps with energy metabolism, eye and skin health
Vitamin B12	Supports new cell development while maintaining nerve cells
Protein	Crucial for building hormones, enzymes and other compounds; provide structure and movement; regulation of body's system; transport
Potassium	Important electrolyte involved with fluid balance and heart health
Vitamin A	Vision, regulation of gene expression, reproduction, bone and tooth growth, immunity

Note: while we discuss cow's milk in this book, because it is where fertility research primarily lends itself, we do understand that for some, cow's milk isn't an option. So we'll talk about the alternatives, too. Here's a quick glance at a few of the most common milk alternatives on the market today so you can see how they compare to cow's milk.

MILK AND MILK ALTERNATIVE NUTRIENT COMPARISON TABLE[21]

	Low-Fat (2%) Cow's Milk + Vitamin A/D	Full-Fat Cow's Milk + Vitamin D	Soymilk, Enriched	Almond Milk	Rice Milk
Serving Size	1 cup	1 cup	1 cup	1 cup	1 cup
Calories	125	150	110	40	115
Total Fat (g)	5	8	5	3	2.5
Saturated Fat (g)	3	5	0	0	0
Cholesterol (mg)	20	24	0	0	0
Sodium (mg)	127	105	122	186	94
Potassium (mg)	446	322	343	176	65
Carbohydrate (g)	12	12	8	1.5	22
Fiber (g)	0	0	1	0	1
Protein (g)	9	8	7	1.6	1
Vitamin A (IU)	500	395	955	372	499
Riboflavin (mg)	.42	.4	.48	.12	.34
Vitamin B12 (mcg)	.93	1.1	2.6	0	1.5
Vitamin D (IU)	98	124	114	110	101
Calcium (mg)	314	276	340	516	283
Phosphorus (mg)	245	205	n/a	26	134

Note: N/A= not available

CHOOSING THE RIGHT DAIRY FOR FERTILITY

Cow's milk is the "gold standard" of milks, in terms of providing the ideal nutrient profile. If you can tolerate cow's milk, consuming three servings may benefit your fertility[22]. That said, the big take home from the longitudinal research is that the *type* of cow's milk you drink actually plays the most significant role in your fertility.

Results from the Nurses Health Study II found that women who consumed more full-fat dairy were less likely to experience ovulatory infertility than those who consumed more low-fat dairy products[13,14]. When looking at the science behind milk and the process that takes place to create the low-fat and skim varieties, we see that a very important component of the milk is altered: the hormones. When the fat is taken away during processing, the ratio of hormones naturally present in the milk is changed, leaving a mix of hormones that isn't ideal for promoting ovulation[13, 14].

When you think about it, it actually makes complete sense. Women who breastfeed produce more of the hormone prolactin, which helps build breast tissue to produce milk. When this occurs, their body changes, and they usually do not ovulate, making conception more of a challenge. Thus, just like a breastfeeding mom, consuming altered portions of hormones through low-fat dairy can affect the body's ovulatory mechanisms.

Although further research has also found that overall dairy intake may increase chances of success in females over thirty-five years old who are undergoing IVF[23], there are conflicting studies where male infertility is concerned. Though limited in size, recent studies do not necessarily support including full-fat dairy in the diets of males who struggle with infertility related to overall sperm quality, or as a means to increase the chance of a successful fertilization when undergoing ART[24, 25].

Now, what should you do? We know it's confusing, but because of the limited sample size of the majority of these studies, we recommend first and foremost discussing this with your doctor. Research supports incorporating one to two servings of whole milk dairy daily while trying to conceive to increase your odds of conception[13, 14]—however, this is contrary to the DGA, as we mentioned above. Personally, we *do* recommend full-fat dairy consumption to females as a means to assist with the complications of ovulatory infertility. We chatted with our physicians and, though they did remind us this is still preliminary research, if we felt better doing so, then we should go for it. However, keep in mind (as indicated above) research does not necessarily support whole milk for males with infertility. Low-fat dairy is speculated to be more conducive to a diet promoting fertility in males. You will see we have included whole milk dairy as the prime base of ingredients in our recipes. However, please note you can easily modify these for your personal dietary needs.

Keep in mind, as well, that whole milk dairy is higher in calories, fat, and saturated fat than its low-fat counterpart. Thus, be mindful of portion sizes to allow yourself the opportunity to fit all foods into a balanced diet to promote your healthiest self. And a gentle reminder, once you *do* conceive (or decide to stop trying), full-fat dairy is not necessarily recommended. Higher saturated fat intakes are linked to a list of other health conditions, such as heart disease.

Bottom line: do what feels best for you and your body, and know that there is evidence to support the benefits of consuming dairy as part of a balanced diet to promote your overall health and well-being, two things we are a hundred percent sure nurture your overall fertility.

PORTION SIZES AND RECIPE RECOMMENDATIONS

The USDA MyPlate Guidelines recommend adults consume up to three one cup (or equivalent) servings of dairy a day[3]. Based on our findings from this research, you'll notice we recommend 1 to 2 servings of full-fat dairy as part of a balanced diet to assist with ovulatory infertility[14]. Rest assured, you will still be able to get adequate calcium in your diet, so no need to worry.

DAIRY FOODS	Amount Equivalent to 1 Serving	Common Portions	Recipe Recommendation
Cow's Milk and Calcium Fortified Soymilk	1 cup milk	1½ string cheese, 1 ounce sliced cheese	*Greek Yogurt Smoothies (page 140)*
Yogurt	8 ounces, 1 cup	6 fluid ounces (most standard containers)	*Sweet Potato Pie Parfait (page 257)*
Cow's Milk Cheese	1½ ounces hard cheese, ⅓ cup shredded cheese, ½ cup cottage cheese, ½ cup ricotta cheese	1½ string cheese, 1 ounce slice sandwich cheese	*Broiled Tomato and Sharp Cheddar Grilled Cheese (page 118)*

PROTEIN

Just like whole grains, proteins come in many shapes and sizes. The common denominator among them is the special "building blocks" known as amino acids. Your body links these amino acids together to build proteins. There are twenty different amino acids that your body needs for making protein, and out of those twenty, there are nine that are considered *essential amino acids*. Your body is unable to make essential amino acids itself, so it relies on you to supply them through the consumption of various foods. (The remaining eleven amino acids are non-essential, because your body is kind enough to make them for you—assuming you eat a variety-filled, balanced diet.) With these amino acids, your body is able to make an incredible array of proteins that carry out an almost endless series of tasks, all without you even realizing it!

Beyond that, protein also supplies your body with energy; however, thanks to carbohydrates and fats, protein is usually reserved for other important functions.

What are those other tasks? Well, how about creating and repairing your body's tissues (bones, muscles, skin and other organs)? That's pretty important. They also act as hormones, antibodies, and enzymes, all of which help our bodies function and heal.

But let's talk a little more about those nine essential amino acids. Those essential amino acids, when available all together in one food source, make what we call a *complete* protein. Basically, that ONE food provides your body with a high-quality protein that readily allows your body to make NEW proteins. Complete proteins are found in animal sources like poultry, beef, pork, fish, dairy, and eggs, as well as vegetarian options such as soy, quinoa, amaranth, buckwheat, hemp seed, and chia seeds. Eating a *variety* of vegetarian foods, like legumes and whole grains, is another way to get all of the amino acids your body needs; that way, even though one food may be missing an amino acid, there's another one that has it. We refer to these as *complementary* proteins.

CHOOSING THE RIGHT PROTEIN FOR FERTILITY

So how do proteins relate to fertility? Findings from the Nurses Health Study II revealed that women who consumed high amounts of animal protein were more likely to experience ovulatory infertility than women who consumed lower amounts of animal proteins. When looking at things closely, the researchers deduced that adding one serving of beans, peas, nuts and peanuts, tofu, or soybeans may actually protect against ovulatory infertility[13,14 26].

Interestingly, one small study suggests that a diet rich in vegetarian protein, specifically soy foods, may be beneficial for women undergoing assisted reproductive therapy[27]. Results revealed that fertilization rates, clinical pregnancies, and live births were all higher among women who consumed more soy foods than those who did not[27]. Other research points to the fact that soy foods may have less of an impact on insulin release than meat foods[13,14]. Too much insulin in the bloodstream has been linked to ovulation problems, including hormonal disruption[13,14].

Our advice? Focus on a diet that includes more plant-based proteins. The possible links to improved fertility are exciting, but so is the research that has proven that consuming a diet rich in fruits, vegetables, whole grains, and nuts and seeds offers seriously great nutrition.

Now, does that mean we're saying not to eat *any* animal proteins? No way! You will soon see we have a great selection of recipes to satisfy our meat eaters in a fertility-fueling way (just take a quick look at the Umami Burger on page 128) or Blackened Shrimp on page 218). Instead, keep your portion sizes in check and balance your meat intake with plenty of vegetables, fruits, nuts, seeds, and whole grains.

PORTION SIZES AND RECIPE RECOMMENDATIONS

The USDA MyPlate Guidelines provide an excellent depiction of just what counts as a serving of protein, since it varies depending on if it's animal- or plant-based. We've included some helpful tips, as well as recipe recommendations, to show you how to apply portion control when it comes to the protein foods. Rest assured, most people get more than enough protein in their daily diets without even having to think about it! We'll chat more in Chapter 3 about just how much your individual body needs (page 51), but take a look below to get you started.

PROTEIN FOODS	Amount Equivalent to 1 Ounce	Common Portions and Ounce Equivalents	Recipe Recommendations
Legumes (Beans, Peas, Soy)	¼ cup of cooked beans (such as black, kidney, pinto, or white beans); ¼ cup of cooked peas (such as chickpeas, lentils, or split peas); ¼ cup (about 2 ounces) of tofu; 2 tablespoons hummus	1 cup bean soup, 1 vegetarian burger, ½ cup beans = 2 ounce equivalents	*Mediterranean Veggie Burger (page 124) or One Pot White Bean and Kale Soup (page 165)*
Nuts and Seeds	½ ounce of nuts (12 almonds, 24 pistachios, 7 walnut halves), ½ ounce of seeds (pumpkin, sunflower, hulled, roasted), 1 tablespoon of nut butter	1 ounce of nuts (¼-⅓ cup, roughly) = 2 ounce equivalents	*Sweet and Spicy Peanuts (page 132)*
Eggs	1 large egg	3 egg whites = 2 ounces, 3 egg yolks = 1 ounce equivalent	*Spinach, Mushroom and Goat Cheese Frittata (page 73)*
Seafood (Fish and Shellfish)	1 ounce cooked fish or shellfish	1 can of tuna/salmon, drained = 3 to 4 ounces, 1 salmon steak = 4 to 6 ounces, 1 small white fish = 3 ounces, 6 large shrimp = 3 ounce equivalents	*Blackened Shrimp (page 218)*

PROTEIN FOODS	Amount Equivalent to 1 Ounce	Common Portions and Ounce Equivalents	Recipe Recommendations
Poultry (Chicken, Turkey)	1 ounce cooked chicken or turkey, without skin 1 sandwich slice of turkey (4½ inches x 2½ inches x ⅛ inches)	1 small chicken breast half = 3 ounce equivalents	*Slow Cooker Pulled Chicken (page 196) or Umami Burger (page 128)*
Red Meat and Pork	1 ounce lean beef or pork	1 small lean hamburger (3 to 4 ounce equivalents)	*Research indicates a plant-based diet is optimal for fertility. Though we don't encourage daily red meat consumption, eating occasionally (1 to 2 times per month) should not inhibit your healthy eating plan, if you so desire.*

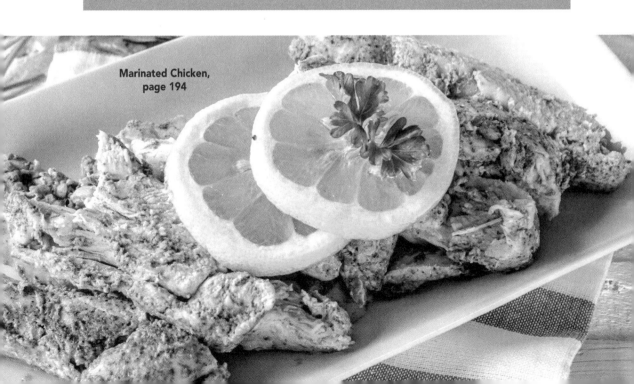

Marinated Chicken, page 194

DIETARY FAT

Fat is fantastic! Yes, you heard us right. This macronutrient has been scrutinized and misunderstood for years. At one point, we were led to believe that fat was the reason we were becoming an overweight society. It plagued us with disease, and so we placed it at the top of the Food Guide Pyramid and encouraged everyone to eat it sparingly. Luckily, we now have evidence that proves not all fat is bad. In fact, fat is *necessary*.

First, it's important to know fat's role in the body. Body fat supplies energy, acting as backup fuel when carbohydrates aren't accessible. Fat acts as a cushion for your organs, helps maintain your body's temperature, and helps mobilize and absorb certain nutrients. Fat is crucial in the development of a baby's brain and nervous system. Plus, adequate body fat is essential for females to menstruate, as well as regulating hormones that are necessary for ovulation (aka, fertility)! On the other hand, excess body fat can actually inhibit ovulation and disrupt your hormonal balance, but we will cover that more in Chapter 3. For now, just remember, fat is *kind of a big deal*.

It's important to know that fats are characterized based on their structure, which consists of *fatty acids* and *glycerol*. The difference in structure is what makes them characteristically different from each other. To make it as simple as possible, take a look at this table. Fertility is complicated enough, fat shouldn't be!

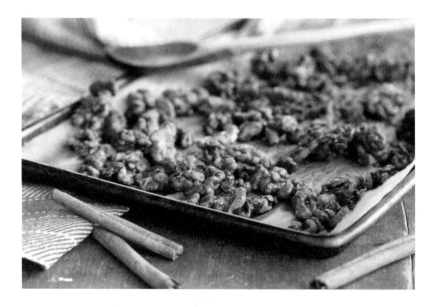

DIETARY FATS

THE "HEALTHY" FATS

Unsaturated Fat:

Where you should get the bulk of your dietary fat

General Traits/Health Impact: Typically liquid at room temperature; can improve total blood cholesterol

Types:

Monounsaturated

Health Impact: Can help decrease total cholesterol and LDL cholesterol

Food Sources: Nuts, avocados, canola oil, olive oil, peanut butter and nuts

Polyunsaturated

Includes two essential fatty acids. The body can't make these fats, so they must be consumed from the diet. A balance between the two is essential. Americans typically have an imbalance, consuming more Omega 6 fatty acids than Omega 3 fatty acids.

Omega 3 Fatty Acids (alpha-linolenic acid)

Health Impact: Can help lower cholesterol, decreasing your risk for heart disease

Food Sources: Salmon, albacore tuna, mackerel, eggs, herring, vegetable oils, flax seed, walnuts

Omega 6 Fatty Acids (linoleic acid)

Health Impact: May promote inflammation

Food Sources: Vegetable oils including corn, safflower, sesame and soy

THE "UNHEALTHY" FATS

Saturated Fat:

Limit your intake and replace with unsaturated fats. The Dietary Guidelines for Americans recommends less than 10 percent of your calories come from saturated fats. Your body makes and utilizes it for various functions, but creates a sufficient amount on its own, so consuming dietary saturated fat isn't warranted.

General Traits/Health Impact: Typically solid at room temperature; large dietary amounts can lead to high cholesterol and high LDL-cholesterol

Food Sources: Meat, poultry, butter, dairy, palm and palm kernel oils, coconut, nuts

Trans Fat:

Limit your intake

General Traits/Health Impact: Can increase total cholesterol and LDL-cholesterol, which negatively impacts cardiovascular health

Food Sources: Found in foods that contain partially hydrogenated oil as well as naturally in meat and dairy products.

CHOOSING THE RIGHT FAT FOR FERTILITY

We've said it before and we'll say it again: fat is your *friend*. But it's important to note what the research says about types of fats and how they affect fertility. Let's take a closer look at current research to clarify our dietary fat recommendations.

First, let's talk about those trans fats. Most research points towards minimizing trans fats from your diet. Go figure, right? A study conducted in 2015 found that higher intakes of trans fats not only affected sperm quality, but also negatively affected gene expression[28]. These findings paralleled a study published in *Human Reproduction* in 2014, which found that men who had higher intakes of trans fats also had lower sperm counts[29].

Though these studies looked specifically at male fertility, it is widely known that higher intakes of trans fat foods can lead to comorbid diseases such as obesity, diabetes, cardio-vascular disease, and hypertension. Because of this, we recommend both males and females minimize their intakes of trans fats from packaged foods. Since dairy and meats naturally contain small portions of trans fat, we do not recommend complete elimination (dairy is crucial for ovulatory infertility), but rather encourage you to be mindful and moderate in your portions.

Now, for the good guys, those unsaturated fatty acids! Without question, poly- and monounsaturated fatty acids are excellent additions to a fertility-fueling diet. You'll notice in the cookbook portion of this book how frequently we rely on monounsaturated fats for a quick salad dressing, sandwich spread, or grab-and-go snack. But the tricky things to navigate are those essential fatty acids, omega-3s and omega-6s.

Research continues to point towards consuming omega-3 rich fish at least twice a week[30]. But the overall ratio of how much omega-3s to omega-6s you should consume varies depending upon which study you look. For instance, a study in 2013 that specifically looked at females undergoing IVF found that higher ratios of omega-6 fatty acids (compared to omega-3 fatty acids) resulted in more favorable odds of embryo implantation[31]. On the other hand, a review conducted in 2007 pointed out that humans now experience higher rates of infertility than in the past[32]. Though not a direct correlation, the researchers highlighted the significant impact the Westernized diet has played on skewing the essential fatty acid ratio from 1:1 (one omega-6 to one omega-3) in the past to the more recent 10:1 ratio[32].

What's our stance? We recommend limiting intakes of saturated and trans fats, relying on wholesome foods prepared with healthy unsaturated fatty acids as the primary source of dietary fat in your diet. You'll see that we include dairy in nearly every recipe in our book, but in small to moderate portions. We also have burgers and other animal-based proteins, but again, these should be eaten in moderation, and combined with vegetables and whole grains to give you the complete nutrient package. Remember, we're showing you how *all* foods can fit in a nutritious, fertility-fueling diet!

PORTION SIZES AND RECIPE RECOMMENDATIONS

The USDA MyPlate Guidelines recommend enjoying healthy fats in moderation, and highlights some of the healthiest choices available. We've included our top selections below, as well as some of the delicious recipes where you can try them. Remember, dietary fat is your friend, and it's important to include it in your daily diet.

Healthy Fat Sources	Standard Serving Amount	Recipe Recommendation
Avocados	1/5 medium (1 ounce)	*No Fail Guacamole (page 116)*
Nut Butters	2 tablespoons	*Natural Peanut Butter (page 59)*
Nuts (Almonds, Cashews, Pecans, Peanuts, Walnuts)	1 ounce	*Roasted Mixed Nuts (page 130)*
Seeds	1 ounce	*Peanut Butter and Banana Toast (page 67)*
Oils (Canola, Olive, Peanut, Sesame, Soybean, Sunflower, Vegetable)	1 tablespoon	*Salad Dressings (page 160)*
Olives	4 olives	*Mediterranean Baked Chicken (page 198)*
Salmon	3 ounces	*Stone-Ground Mustard and Apricot Glazed Salmon (page 214)*

OTHER NUTRIENTS TO CONSIDER
CALCIUM

According to the 2015 Dietary Guidelines for Americans, calcium is an under-consumed nutrient, despite the recommendation of three servings of dairy per day[33]. Even though one to two servings of whole milk dairy are recommended daily to assist with ovulatory infertility, there are other food sources of dietary calcium you can include, as well. Here's a list of calcium-rich foods, along with recipes to try from the cookbook.

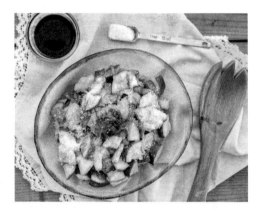

Food	Recipe Recommendation
Arugula	Arugula Salad with Apricots and Champagne Vinaigrette (page 147)
Broccoli	Broccoli Cheese Soup (page 173)
Cheese	Broiled Tomato and Sharp Cheddar Grilled Cheese (page 118)
Legumes	One Pot White Bean and Kale Soup (page 165)
Sesame Seed	Tahini Vinaigrette (page 163)
Spinach	Garlic Spinach with Sliced Almonds (page 227)
Tofu	Stir Fry Tofu (page 206)
Whole Grains	Light and Fluffy Whole Wheat Pancakes (page 89), Whole Wheat Freezer Waffles (page 92)

Dietary Reference Intake: 1000 mg/day (Refer to Appendix, page 267)

FOLATE (FOLIC ACID)

Folate (vitamin B9) is an essential B vitamin, necessary for creating and maintaining healthy red blood cells. Folate refers to the vitamin found in food and our bodies, while folic acid is the synthetic version provided through supplements and fortified foods. Interestingly, folic acid is more readily absorbed by your body than folate. To account for these discrepancies and to ensure you're getting enough of this important vitamin when evaluating your diet, folate intake

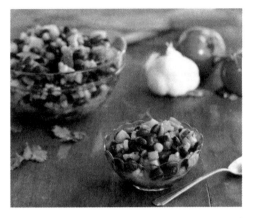

can be expressed in Dietary Folate Equivalents (DFE). These conversions allow you and your health practitioners to assess if your folate intake is adequate. For reference, use the following conversions.

FOLATE (MCG)	DIETARY FOLATE EQUIVALENTS (DFE)
Food Folate: 1 mcg	1 DFE
Synthetic Folate (folic acid): 1 mcg	1.7 DFE

It's no wonder countless advertisements and research studies tout the importance of having adequate folate when trying to conceive, since this is one vitamin that is essential in building new life. The Nurses Health Study II even indicated that women who received at least 700 mcg of folic acid per day were 40 to 50 percent less likely to experience ovulatory infertility than those who consumed less than 300 mg[13,14]. The recommended dietary intakes (DRI) for folate are 400 mcg per day (see Appendix page 267); however, with conception and pregnancy, those needs increase to 600 mcg per day, or possibly up to 800 mcg per day, depending on your reproductive endocrinologist's recommendations. Get a jump start on increasing your dietary folate intake by incorporating more of the following foods, and talk to your doctor about taking a daily prenatal multivitamin.

Food	Recipe Recommendation
Avocado	No Fail Guacamole (page 116)
Beans, Legumes	Black Bean Salad with Honey-Lime Vinaigrette (page 152)
Beets	Jalapeno Beet Hummus (page 104)
Enriched Cereal	Breakfast Choices (page 56)
Spinach	Spinach, Mushroom and Goat Cheese Frittata (page 73)

Dietary Reference Intake: 400 mcg/day (Refer to Appendix, page 267)

IRON

Iron is a trace mineral with an important job. As part of hemoglobin, iron carries oxygen in our blood, where it is distributed throughout our cells to be used for energy production. It also serves an important role in immunity and brain development. Low iron stores can lead to a condition called anemia, or "too little blood." A lack of iron 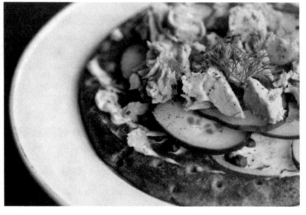 equates to a lack of oxygen, which can impair energy levels, as well as a host of other symptoms.

Iron can be found in both animal (heme) and plant (nonheme) sources. And while it's plentiful in terms of availability, our bodies don't always absorb it. Why? One reason is because of the difference between heme and nonheme iron. Heme iron is more readily absorbed by the body than nonheme iron. Also, certain foods can actually increase or decrease your body's absorption of both heme and nonheme iron. See our handy chart below.

INCREASES IRON ABSORPTION	DECREASES IRON ABSORPTION
Vitamin C	Chocolate and spinach (oxalic acid)
Meat, fish, poultry (MFP factor*)	Tea, coffee (tannins)
Cooking with cast iron	Calcium and phosphorus (milk, dairy)
	Legumes, whole grain cereals (phytates)

* MFP factor: found in meat, poultry and fish, and helps with the absorption of nonheme iron when eaten with non-heme iron foods.

You know from our protein discussion that plant based proteins are highly encouraged in a fertility-fueling diet. That's why it's important to create balance and include plenty of variety. Here's a list of iron-rich foods (and related recipes) to include in your diet to boost your iron levels.

Food Source	Recipe Recommendation
Beans, Legumes	*White Bean and Rosemary Spread (page 107), Red Lentil Curry Soup (page 168)*
Chicken	*Slow Cooker Pulled Chicken (page 196)*
Kale	*Lacinato Kale Salad with Peaches and Maple Vinaigrette (page 154)*
Salmon	*Stone-Ground Mustard and Apricot Glazed Salmon (page 214)*
Spinach	*Parmesan Pesto Pasta with Cherry Tomatoes (page 183)*
Whole Grains (Quinoa)	*Protein Packed Freezer Burritos (page 212)*

Dietary Reference Intake: 18 mg/day (Refer to Appendix, page 267)

SELENIUM

Another trace mineral that shows promise in terms of male infertility is selenium. Though research is still preliminary, one study found that selenium, when paired with Vitamin E, may improve sperm motility and morphology[34]. Selenium acts as an antioxidant, protecting our bodies against oxidative damage. Partnering with vitamin E, selenium comes to the rescue to rid our bodies of free radicals (those bad guys we chatted about on page 12) that may have the ability to inhibit fertility. Include the foods below to boost your selenium intake, as your need for this nutrient only increases once you become pregnant.

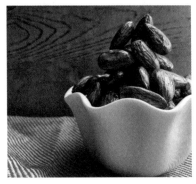

Food	Recipe Recommendation
Brazil Nuts	Roasted Mixed Nuts (page 130)
Chicken	Chicken Salad Wrap (page 122)
Mushrooms	Parmesan Portobello Burger (page 126)
Vegetables and Whole Grains (soil dependent)	Roasted Vegetables (page 223)
Shellfish	Blackened Shrimp (page 218)

Dietary Reference Intake: 55 mg/day (Refer to Appendix, page 267)

VITAMIN D

The "sunshine vitamin" is getting a lot of attention these days because of the fact that countless Americans are deficient. Vitamin D is essential for regulating blood calcium and ensuring our bones remain strong. In addition, Vitamin D is the only vitamin that is converted into a hormone to act as a messenger, allowing the body's cells to communicate with each other. As you can imagine, having cells communicate properly is crucial for conception.

Also of note, a recent study found that women deficient in vitamin D while undergoing IVF saw a decrease in their chance of success[35].

While we aren't recommending supplementation, we do encourage you to get your vitamin D levels tested and speak with your physician about the right plan for you. In the meantime, here are some Vitamin D-rich foods to focus on in your diet.

Food Source	Recipe Recommendations
Enriched Cereal	Homemade Granola Bars (page 136)
Fortified Milk, Juice	Strawberry Banana Smoothie (page 140)
Salmon	Stone Ground Mustard and Apricot Glazed Salmon (page 214)
Sunlight	Natural sunlight promotes vitamin D synthesis in the skin!

Dietary Reference Intake: 600 IU/day (Refer to Appendix, page 267)

ZINC

Zinc is a trace mineral that is essential for normal ovulation as well as sperm production—primary concerns for those struggling with ovulatory and male infertility. Zinc is in many of the fertility-fueling foods you'll find through our cookbook, such as in the following:

Food	Recipe Recommendations
Dairy (yogurt)	Sweet Potato Pie Parfait (page 257)
Meat (Chicken, Fish, Turkey)	Umami Burger (page 128)
Whole Grains	Sesame Whole Wheat Noodles (page 240)

Dietary Reference Intake: 8 mg/day (Refer to Appendix, page 267)

CHOLINE

Choline is an essential micronutrient that is vital for many functions in the body, including metabolism, memory, physical activity, and maintaining heart health. However, choline is also crucial for those trying to conceive and mothers who become pregnant because it not only builds the foundation for a healthy brain, but also helps prevent neural tube defects. Choline is not found in prenatal vitamins, so make the most of what you're eating to get your recommended 425 mg per day (450 mg per day if pregnant). Here are some ways to help increase your choline intakes through your diet:

Food	Recipe Recommendations
Eggs	*Kimchi Baked Eggs (page 74)*
Meat (Chicken, Fish, Turkey)	*Stone Ground Mustard and Apricot Glazed Salmon (page 214)*
Green Vegetables (Spinach, Kale)	*Garlic Spinach with Sliced Almonds (page 227)*

Dietary Reference Intake: 425 mg/day (Refer to Appendix, page 267)

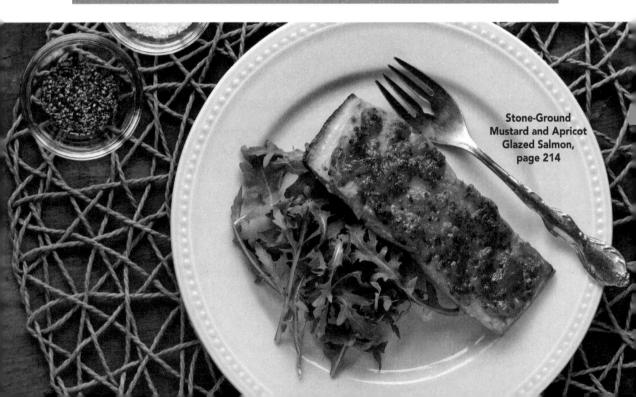

Stone-Ground Mustard and Apricot Glazed Salmon, page 214

PUTTING YOUR PLATE TOGETHER

Now that you've mastered the food groups, it's time to learn how to put it all together. Thankfully, that's as easy as following the MyPlate guidelines.

You'll notice that we don't address calories much here. That's by design; while we appreciate the value of calories, we don't appreciate the concept of calorie counting. From our experience, counting calories is a dated practice that's overwhelming and unnecessary. But we know understanding daily caloric needs can be helpful when learning how to incorporate MyPlate into your life. Just remember, every person has individual nutrition needs that vary based on activity levels, medical history, and weight. Registered dietitian nutritionists often rely on the Harris Benedict Equation (cited below) to estimate one's daily needs.

CALCULATING DAILY NEEDS	
REE (RESTING ENERGY EXPENDITURE)	
WT. IN KG = POUNDS/2.2 ; HT. IN CM = INCHES X 2.54	
Males	65.5 + 13.75 (wt. in kg) + 5.0 (ht. in cm) - 6.78 (age in years)
Females	655 + 9.56 (wt. in kg) + 1.85 (ht. in cm) - 4.68 (age in years)

The best recommendation is to seek the help of a registered dietitian nutritionist who can help you understand your needs, then use the table below as a guide based on your daily needs. For a specific look at Dietary Reference Intakes (DRIs), take a look at the DRI charts (page 267).

MYPLATE DAILY RECOMMENDED SERVINGS PER FOOD GROUP[3]

Food Group	1600 Calorie	1800 Calorie	2000 Calorie	2200 Calorie
Grains	5 ounces	6 ounces	6 ounces	7 ounces
Protein	5 ounces	5 ounces	5½ ounces	6 ounces
Fruits	1½ cups	1½ cups	2 cups	2 cups
Vegetables	2 cups	2½ cups	2½ cups	3 cups
Dairy	3 cups	3 cups	3 cups	3 cups
Fat	Use sparingly			

We recommend taking a prenatal MVI (multivitamin) daily as a "safety net" to ensure your nutritional needs are met.

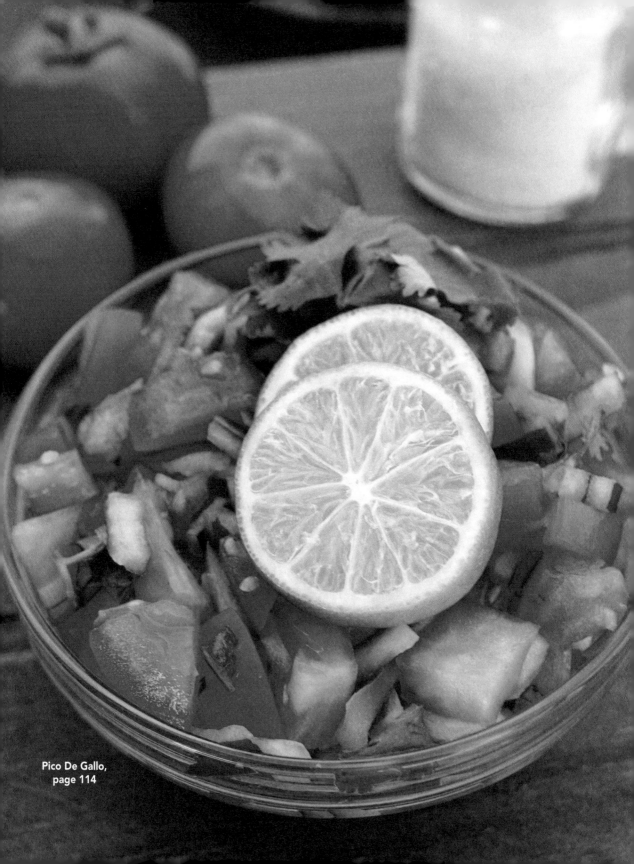

Pico De Gallo,
page 114

Chapter 3

The Secondary Ingredients—Other Fertility Factors

LIFESTYLE FACTORS

What's the first thing you did when you found out you were struggling with infertility? We can tell you ours. We can't say we're *proud*, but it shows you we're human, too:

> Sara: I was mad. I was flat-out *angry* about being "infertile." Fueling that anger were the constant reminders of my infertility—every day was a new challenge, because I felt like I was surrounded by babies and pregnant women. It didn't matter where I was, whether it was the train or at the store, I felt those little cherub faces looking at me and those big, ripe, pregnant bellies figuratively, and sometimes literally, bumping me. I felt so sorry for myself. I was certain they hadn't struggled like me. They were probably like every other woman I know, who just *blinked* and got pregnant. So, yes, I was angry, and I allowed myself to *be* angry.
>
> But that could only last so long. I decided I'd had enough and turned towards that Bigger Power with prayer. Prayer led me to peace, and that peace led me to the bookstore, where I found great books, such as Alice Domar's *Conquering Infertility*, that helped me deal with the emotional side of this infertility journey. From those books, I found the tools I needed to help me cope when those little baby faces and pregnant bellies got to be too much.

Liz: Since I feel like getting my official diagnosis of infertility took almost two years, I equate it to slowly pulling off hot wax from your leg. Sure, it's easier to do in one quick pull, but sometimes you go hair by hair, feeling the pain with every tug. I remember how, when it all started, I felt so alone. So scared. Sure, my husband was great, but he didn't know what I was feeling. I threw my love for morning coffee out the window, amped up my veggies, and stopped working out. I was positive that would click the switch.

I also considered getting a dog. Sure, my husband is allergic to pet hair and I myself am just not an animal person, but I thought it would fill that void. Thankfully, I snapped out of it before my husband came home to find a puppy in the house. But, it goes to show that irrational impulses happen to all of us when we desire to find control.

We both felt alone, out of control, and restless. We sought comfort, and we recognized nutrition could provide it for us. We embarked on a journey to conquer a wholesome, nutrient-dense meal plan, fueling our bodies with foods that would make us feel our best, both inside and out.

While we certainly aren't suggesting you cut out any foods from your diet, we do want to point out how certain diet and lifestyle factors can actually *hurt* your fertility. It may seem obvious to some, but in all fairness it's news to many: tobacco use, alcohol consumption, and drugs will significantly and negatively impact your fertility. If you engage in any of these behaviors, it's important to remove them from your lifestyle before trying to conceive. We recommend speaking with a health professional who specializes in this area for the best support. The good news is that from speaking with licensed psychologist Dr. Jeff Daly, we can confirm that there are immediate and long term physical and psychological benefits of substance cessation that can promote both fertility and conception. (Please see our list of resources on page 279 for your reference.)

BODY WEIGHT AND FITNESS: WHAT'S APPROPRIATE?

There are two different sides to the weight issue when considering infertility. Being over-weight or underweight can both significantly affect your chances of conception. Eating disorders and disordered eating behaviors often coincide with infertility. If you struggle with a diagnosed eating disorder or disordered eating behaviors, we recommend that you immediately seek help. Please see the appendix for resources to guide you (page 265). This book is only a piece of the puzzle for you, and there are many excellent resources to help you on the journey to attaining a nutrient-dense diet.

Body weight, in terms of exact numbers, is not the sole tool we as registered dietitian nutritionists use to quantify health. We know that body composition (your ratio of body fat to muscle) is a much more valid measure of determining your health. However, many health professionals still use body mass index (BMI) to diagnose an individual as overweight, normal weight, or underweight. Though we don't necessarily agree with it for this purpose, we have included here as a reference, as you've likely heard (or will hear) these terms in your appointments.

BMI (BODY MASS INDEX) Formula: weight (lb.)/[height(in)]² x 703	
Classification	**BMI**
Underweight	<18.5
Normal weight	**18.4 to 24.9**
Overweight	**25 to 29.9**
Obese	**>30**

If your weight is a concern, there are changes you can make that will increase your fertility. If you are overweight, beginning an exercise regimen (with your doctor's approval) along with following the nutrition recommendations in this book (and the additional assistance from a registered dietitian nutritionist) will lead to improved cardiovascular health and help lower your total body fat, ultimately making your body healthier to accept conception.

If you are underweight, focusing on fueling your body with nutrient-dense foods, including healthy fats found in foods like avocados, nuts, and full fat dairy, will help to increase your body weight without making you feel sluggish.

While it's important to limit your strenuous activity if you are an active athlete, it is also important to find balance. We both gave up exercise as a means to control our fertility odds, and it left us feeling irritated, angry, and upset. If you love running, there's no need to hang up your running shoes—just loosen the laces a little bit!

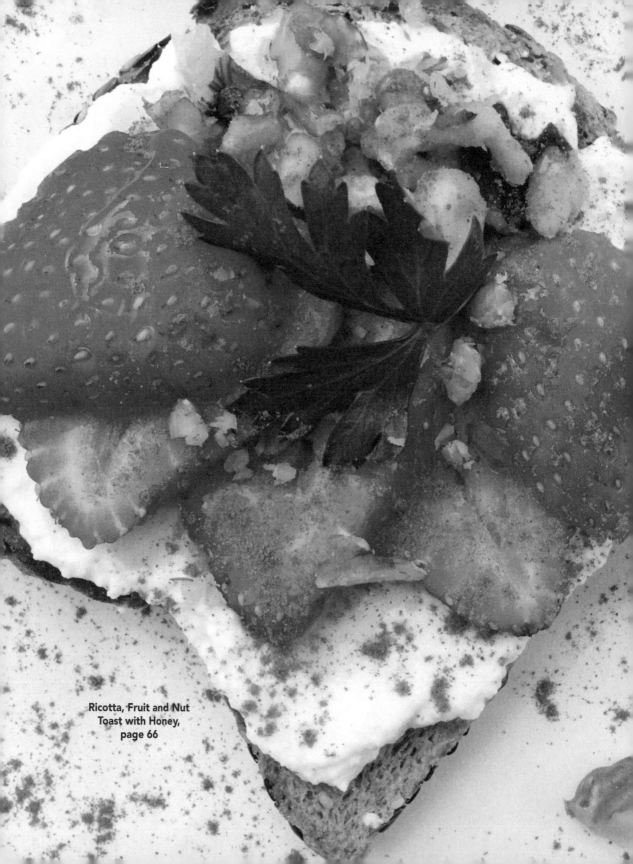

Ricotta, Fruit and Nut
Toast with Honey,
page 66

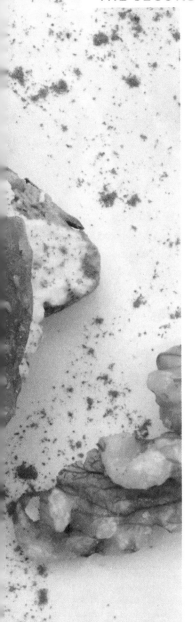

In the end, we encourage finding a routine that works best for you. Instead of strenuous exercise, consider other means of physical activity that can provide an outlet for stress and anxiety. We encourage you to take a look at the strategies below, cited from a personal interview with Dana Peters, MA, Life Coach.

ALTERNATIVE COPING STRATEGIES FOR MANAGING STRESS

- Find a support network (online or in your community)

- Yoga

- Listen to music

- Paint or do something artistic

- Call a friend

- Find a scented candle you enjoy and light it when you feel anxious or depressed

- Distract yourself with an activity, such as crocheting or knitting

- Sip hot tea

- Pet your dog, cat or other pet

- Clean your house or organize your closet

- Take a bubble bath

- Watch your favorite funny movie or read a book you enjoy

- Journal

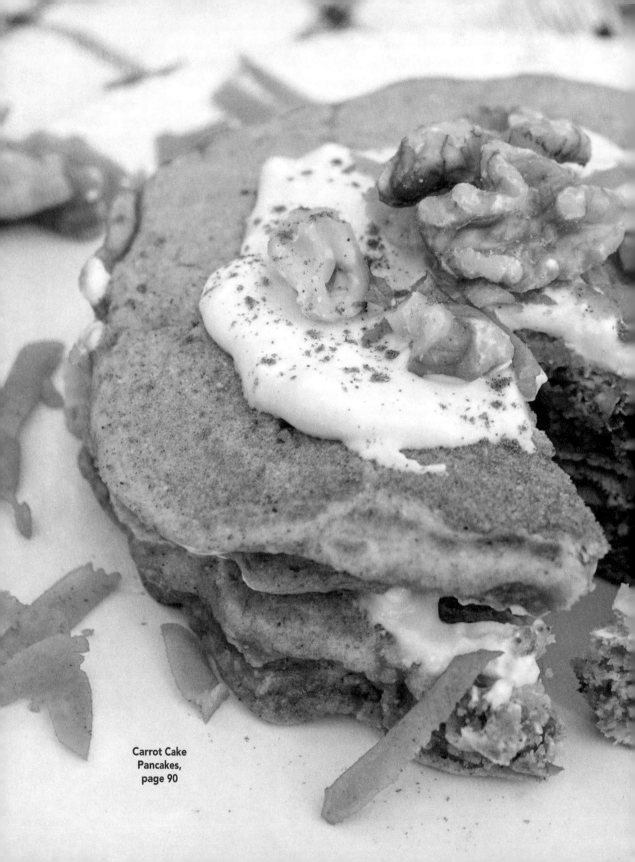

Carrot Cake
Pancakes,
page 90

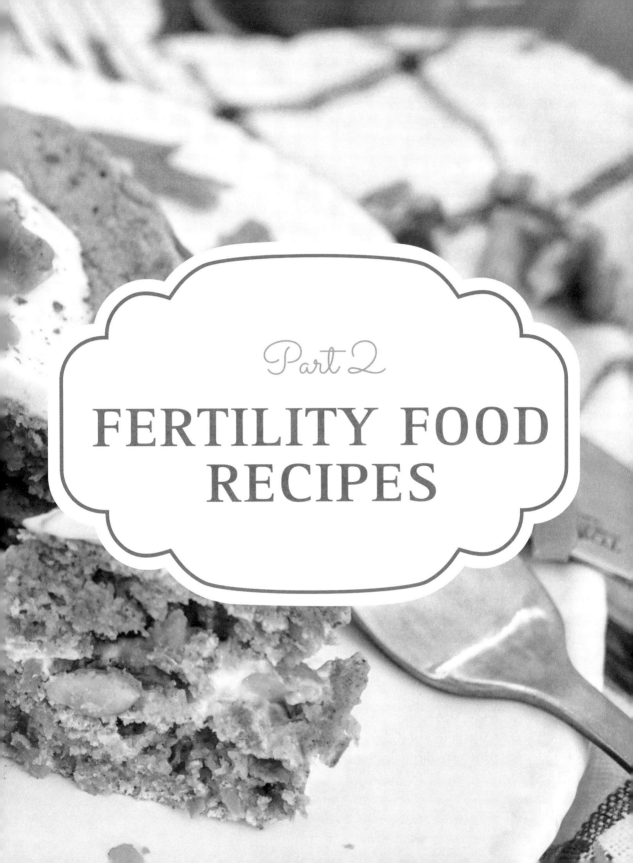

Part 2

FERTILITY FOOD RECIPES

*A*re you ready for those delicious recipes we promised you?
Now it's time to apply what you've learned so that you can begin to nourish your body and mind. Our goal is to take the guesswork out of meal planning, providing recipes and showing you what foods pair together in a synergistic relationship to help fuel your fertility and give you the energy to feel your best. But before we jump in, let's review first and foremost *how* to read a recipe, followed by the important basics when it comes to cooking and food safety.

HOW TO READ THE RECIPES

Have you ever started making a recipe, and everything was going well until, all of a sudden, it wasn't? Out of nowhere, the recipe calls for chopped onion and you don't have any. You scramble to cut the onion while the pan on the stove is about ready to burn your chicken and the timer is going off to alert you that your broccoli is done roasting. Ugh! No wonder you don't like cooking. But what if we told you there's a way to prevent this kitchen conundrum? Well, rest assured, there is! Better yet, we're going to ease your stress and anxiety with three simple tips that will help you master any recipe.

Tip 1) Read the recipe first. Yes, it's that simple! Would you assemble a piece of furniture without first reading the instructions? No way! Well, recipes are no different. It's imperative that you read all of the steps so that you are prepared when you start cooking. This is how you take the anxiety out of cooking!

Tip 2) *Mis en place.* So French, but oh, so important! *Mis en place* literally translates to "everything in its place." It means that *after* you read the recipe and *before* you start cooking, you prep all of your ingredients and get yourself organized. This is the time to chop that onion, rinse those beans, or complete whatever task you need to before you start cooking. This will save you time and sanity, trust us!

Tip 3) Know the terms. *Sear, sauté, simmer*—what do they all mean? If you don't know, it's okay. Since you've read the recipe *before* you started cooking, you have time to figure that out. And lucky for you, we've included a table in the Appendices that explains all of these cooking techniques so that you don't have to be confused.

RECIPE KEY

Finally, the recipes! We're going to challenge you to think outside of the box here, friends!
We chatted with wannabe mothers and mothers struggling with secondary infertility to learn just what foods they enjoy most so that we could highlight the best of the best in

these recipes. We want to show you how your familiar foods can be incorporated into a fertility-fueling diet, while also introducing you to some new ideas that may just become your *new* favorites! After you've perused the recipes, check out the shopping list we've developed to help make your life a little easier (pages 269–272). We all could use a bit more *easy* in our lives, right?

SERVINGS AND DIETARY ACCOMMODATIONS

Most recipes are designed to yield 4 to 8 servings so that you can embrace the joy of leftovers. And since we know that there are dietary restrictions and lifestyle preferences that will require recipe modifications, we've listed the allergens below all the nutrition facts, as well as whether the recipe is gluten free, vegan, or vegetarian.

For most recipes, a plant based milk alternative can be used in place of whole milk for a vegan option. Or, if you're looking to assist with male infertility, a low-fat dairy product can be used as well in place of the whole milk suggestions. In addition, a gluten-free flour blend can be used in place of the whole grain flour. These have not been tested, though, so please note to proceed with caution. However, we will reiterate that, unless medically necessitated, the research *does* lend support to the use of whole milk in facilitating the most optimal fertility environment.

For recipes that can be made gluten free or vegan, we've used the indication, "* = Gluten Free/Vegan Option". If you have a medical condition, such as celiac disease, lactose intolerance, food allergies, or another similar condition, we recommend you speak with a registered dietitian nutritionist to design the plan that works best with your nutrition needs. See Appendix (page 279) for references.

MYPLATE KEY

We told you we wanted to personalize this book for you! Throughout the recipe collection we use the following icons to indicate how each recipe meets your MyPlate needs.

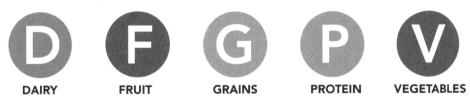

For instance: see how the Grecian Grain Bowl (page 208) boasts not only whole grains, but also has protein, vegetables, and dairy.

NUTRITION FACTS

Each recipe contains the following nutrition facts information, analyzed using The Food Processor:

NUTRITION INFORMATION

PER SERVING: Calories xx; Fat xx g (Sat xx g); Protein xx g; Carb xx g; Fiber xx g; Calcium xx mg; Iron xx mg; Sodium xx mg; Folate xx mcg

---

Please note that, since added sugars are not nutritionally the same as natural sugars, we have omitted this value. Our focus is to show you how you can maximize your nutrition and use wholesome ingredients to create nutrient-dense meals to fuel your fertility. Thus, a majority of sugar sources used in the recipes are naturally-based. For more information on how each recipe meets your daily reference intakes, refer to the appendix DRI charts (page 267).

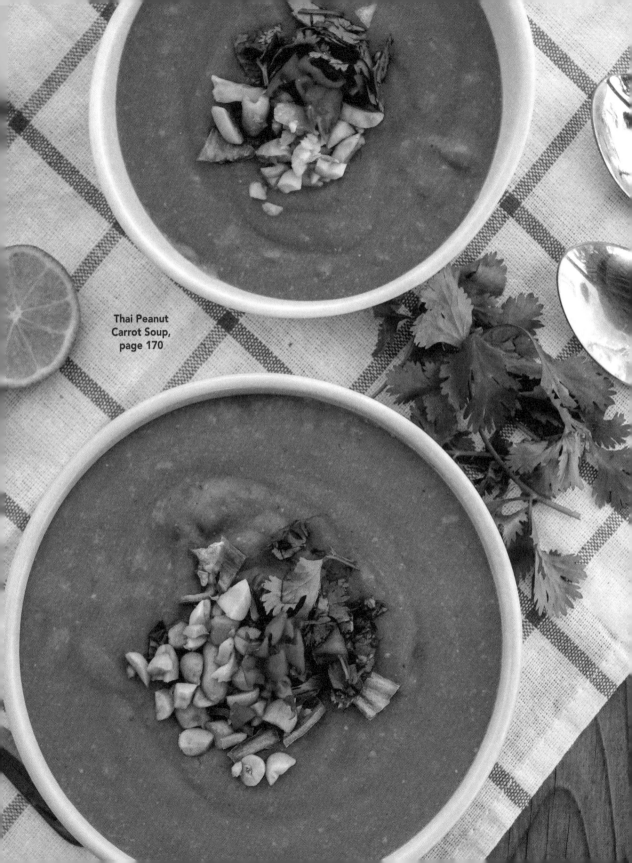

Thai Peanut
Carrot Soup,
page 170

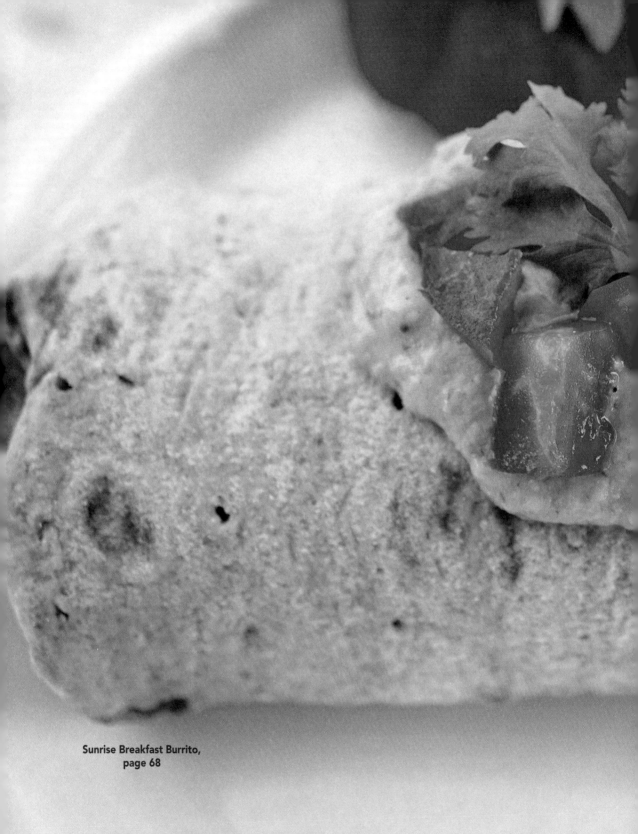
Sunrise Breakfast Burrito,
page 68

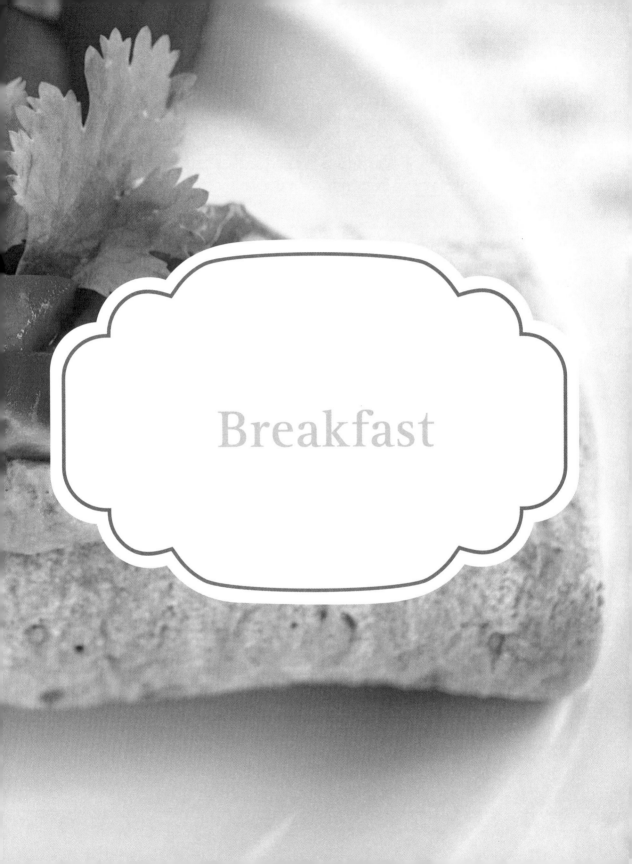

Breakfast

BREAKFAST IS ONE OF the most important meals of your day! Not only are you *breaking* the *fast* from your eight hours (hopefully!) of slumber, but you're also refueling your tank to power you through your morning. We understand how difficult it can be to think about finding creative ways to nourish your body this early in the morning. Plus, we also suggest you switch from a large coffee to a small one, which for many can be a tough transition.

To help you ease into these changes, we've come up with a list of breakfast basics to give you the nutritional boost your body needs. These recipes don't require endless hours in the kitchen—we know you don't have that! So rest assured: with a little bit of meal prep, you can easily whip these dishes up and be out the door in no time.

And for those days when you really feel yourself dragging, here's a list of simple, no-fuss breakfast ideas to fuel your fertility, too!

STAPLE FOOD	ENHANCE WITH THESE FERTILITY FOODS
Scrambled Eggs	Diced or chopped mushrooms or bell peppers, whole milk cheese, black beans
Hard Boiled Egg	Mix with 2 tablespoons 4 percent fat large curd cottage cheese, black pepper, kosher salt and top on avocado toast
Whole Milk Greek Yogurt	Fruit (fresh or unsweetened frozen or canned), chia seeds, walnuts
Smoothie	1 cup whole milk or whole milk yogurt base, ½ cup frozen berries
Steel Cut or Rolled Oats	¾ cup whole milk, 1 tablespoon chopped walnuts, ½ cup fresh fruit
Whole Grain Cereal	Choose a cereal with less than 5 grams sugar, more than 4 grams fiber and made with whole grains
Whole Grain Toast	Top with 1 tablespoon nut or seed butter, along with 1 teaspoon of jelly or jam of your choice

All Natural Berry Jam

(F) **MAKES: 1 cup, 16 servings, 1 tablespoon each**
GLUTEN FREE, VEGETARIAN

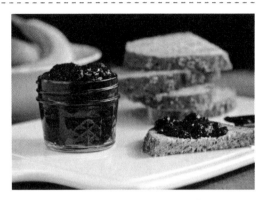

The secret to this jam's success? Chia seeds! Not only do they thicken the jam and add texture, they're also an excellent source of omega-3 fatty acids. This jam tastes great as the jelly for the PB&J Greek Yogurt Parfaits (page 82). If you like the texture of a seedy jam, this recipe is for you!

1 tablespoon honey
¼ cup orange juice
1 cup fresh or frozen berries of your choice
1 cup strawberries, hulled and quartered
2 tablespoons chia seeds
1 teaspoon orange zest

Combine the honey and orange juice in a small saucepan and bring to a boil over medium heat. Add the berries, then reduce the heat to medium-low and simmer uncovered, stirring occasionally, for about 20 minutes.

Remove saucepan from the heat and mash gently with a spoon. Stir in the chia seeds. Allow mixture to cool, then add the orange zest. Transfer the jam to a clean bowl and/or jar and cover with a clean lid. Refrigerate until ready to enjoy.

Storage: Jam needs to be refrigerated in an airtight container and enjoyed within 2 weeks.

Kitchen Tip: If using frozen berries, you may need to add additional chia seeds to thicken the mixture. Add 1 teaspoon at a time until desired consistency is reached.

NUTRITION INFORMATION
PER SERVING: Calories 25; Fat 0.5g (Sat 0g); Protein 1g; Carb 4g; Fiber 1g; Calcium 13mg; Iron 0.2mg; Sodium 5mg; Folate 4mcg

---

FERTILITY FOCUS: Chia seeds are a great source of omega-3 fatty acids, which are crucial for heart health and fetal brain development. By incorporating chia seeds into everyday foods, you can easily boost your intake of this nutritious type of fat!

Zesty Lime Mango Preserves

 MAKES: ¾ cup, 12 servings, 1 tablespoon each
GLUTEN FREE, VEGAN

Making your own preserves is easy, and the result is a delicious spread with endless possibilities! Use this as a fun topping for Toasted Coconut Waffles (page 94).

2 cups ¼-inch chopped fresh
    or frozen mango (about 12 ounces
    or 2 mangos)
2 tablespoons granulated sugar
1 tablespoon lemon or lime juice
¼ teaspoon lime zest

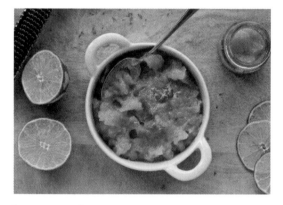

NUTRITION INFORMATION
PER SERVING: Calories 25; Fat 0g (Sat 0g); Protein 0g; Carb 10g; Fiber 0g; Calcium 3mg; Iron 0.1mg; Sodium 0mg; Folate 12mcg

Place all ingredients except zest in a small saucepan. Bring to a boil over medium-high heat.

Reduce heat to medium-low and simmer, stirring occasionally, for about 20 to 30 minutes or until thickened slightly. Mash mango with a potato masher or the back of a fork to create a smoother consistency.

Remove from heat and allow preserves to cool before stirring in lime zest and placing in a clean jar or bowl. Once fully cooled, cover with a clean lid or plastic wrap and refrigerate.

Storage: Preserves need to be refrigerated in an airtight container and enjoyed within 7 to 10 days.

FERTILITY FOCUS: We know that a healthy weight is important when it comes to fertility. Too much added sugar (defined as more than ten percent of daily calories) is not beneficial to a fertility fueling diet. That's why these preserves only use 2 tablespoons of granulated sugar in the whole recipe!

Natural Peanut Butter

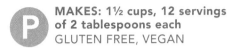

P **MAKES: 1½ cups, 12 servings of 2 tablespoons each**
GLUTEN FREE, VEGAN

Plant-based proteins, like peanuts, are a great way to help curb your appetite and keep you feeling satisfied until your next eating occasion. Try this nut butter on Whole Wheat Freezer Waffles (page 92) or as a simple snack with fresh fruit!

16 ounces dry roasted peanuts, unsalted
¾ teaspoon kosher salt

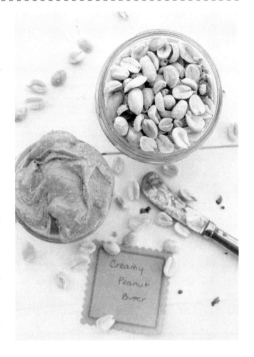

Add peanuts to the bowl of a food processor and process on low speed for 2 minutes. Using a spatula, scrape down the sides of the bowl, replace top and continue to process on low for 2 to 3 minutes. Add salt and pulse another minute or until desired consistency is reached. Transfer to a jar with a lid and store in the refrigerator.

Variation: Roasted almonds or walnuts can be used in place of peanuts. Processing times may vary depending on nut and desired consistency.

Storage: Store in a sealed jar in the refrigerator and use within 2 months.

NUTRITION INFORMATION
PER SERVING: Calories 220; Fat 19g (Sat 3g); Protein 9g; Carb 8g; Fiber 3g; Calcium 22mg; Iron 0.6mg; Sodium 150mg; Folate 37mcg
ALLERGENS: Peanuts (or tree nuts for variation)

FERTILITY FOCUS: Nut butters are a great source of nutrition, including heart-healthy fats and proteins. This simple DIY peanut butter also boasts antioxidant power, making it a fantastic fuel for fertility.

Vanilla (or Cocoa) Cinnamon Nut Butter

MAKES: 1¼ cups, 20 servings, 1 tablespoon each
GLUTEN FREE, VEGAN

Nut butter's dessert-style twin Cookie Butter gets a makeover with this healthy, no-added-sugar version. This nut butter tastes wonderful as a sweet addition to sliced apples, or spread over Light and Fluffy Whole Wheat Pancakes (page 89)!

½ cup Natural Peanut Butter (page 59) or store bought natural peanut butter
1 cup roasted almonds
1 teaspoon vanilla extract
1 teaspoon ground cinnamon

In the bowl of a food processor, add the peanut butter, almonds, vanilla extract, and ground cinnamon, and process on low speed for 1 minute. Scrape down sides of processor with a spatula and process one more minute. If you prefer a smoother texture, process for an additional minute. Transfer to a jar with a lid and store in the refrigerator.

Variation: To make Chocolate Cookie Butter, add 1½ teaspoons of unsweetened cocoa powder along with the cinnamon.

Storage: Store in a sealed jar in the refrigerator and use within 2 months.

NUTRITION INFORMATION
PER SERVING: Calories 90; Fat 8g (Sat 1g); Protein 3; Carb 3g; Fiber 1g; Calcium 23mg; Iron 0.4mg; Sodium 30mg; Folate 11mcg
ALLERGENS: Peanuts, Tree Nuts

FERTILITY FOCUS: It's important to keep the amount of added sugar you eat to a minimum, because too much added sugar can increase circulating blood sugar. Studies have shown an elevated blood sugar level may increase the odds of infertility.

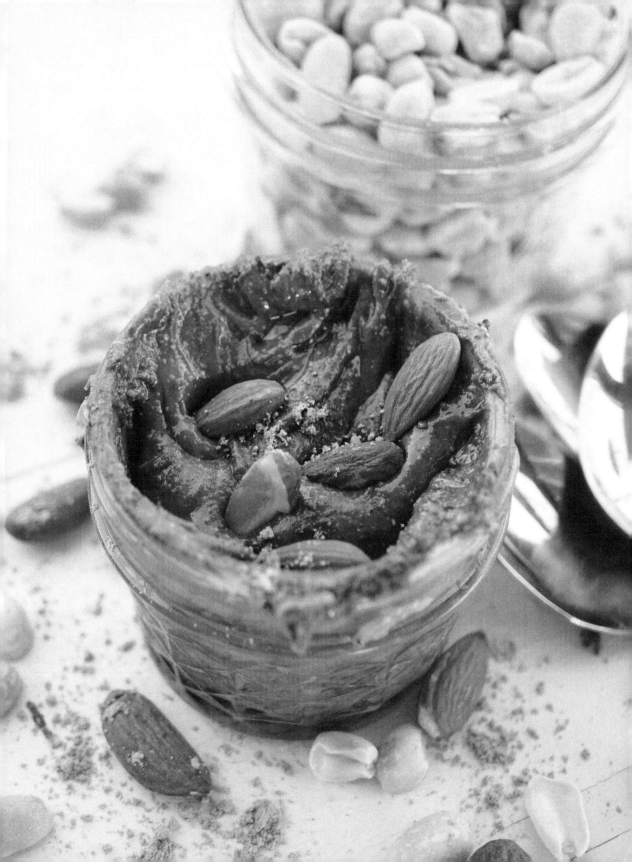

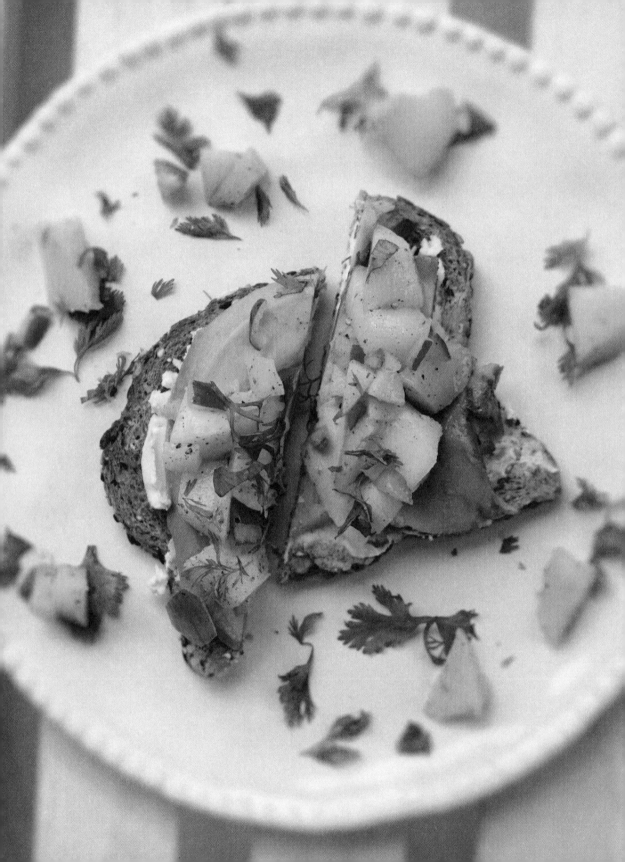

Tropical Toast with a Cayenne Kick

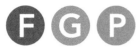

MAKES: 1 serving
GLUTEN FREE*, VEGETARIAN

Toast is trendy! This recipe, and the ones that follow, show how you can upgrade your traditional toast into a fertility-fueling meal. These toasts are packed with whole grains, protein, fruit, and dairy. Feel free to substitute a gluten free bread of your choice, if desired. This recipe lets you spice up your morning toast with a zesty kick of cayenne and fresh mango!

1 slice (1½ ounces) whole grain
 bread^{GF}
3 tablespoons (¾ ounce) finely
 chopped fresh mango
2 teaspoons red onion, finely diced
¼ teaspoon cayenne pepper
½ teaspoon fresh lime juice
2 tablespoons (½ ounce) goat
 cheese
⅕ medium (1 ounce) avocado,
 thinly sliced
¼ teaspoon ground black pepper
⅛ teaspoon kosher salt
2 teaspoons fresh cilantro, chopped

Toast the bread. Combine mango and red onion in a bowl along with the cayenne pepper and lime juice. Spread goat cheese on top of the toasted bread and top with sliced avocado and mango mixture. Sprinkle with pepper and salt, and garnish with chopped cilantro.

NUTRITION INFORMATION
PER SERVING: Calories 250; Fat 10g (Sat 4.5g); Protein 12g; Carb 30g; Fiber 6g; Calcium 194mg; Iron 1.8mg; Sodium 510mg; Folate 57mcg
ALLERGENS: Wheat, Milk
* = Gluten Free Option

FERTILITY FOCUS: Enjoying avocado as a part of a balanced diet is a great way to boost your intake of unsaturated fat. This form of good-for-you fat helps satisfy and, when eaten in place of saturated or trans fats, also keeps your heart healthy. What mom-to-be doesn't need a strong ticker?

Ricotta Pesto Toast with Walnuts and Tomatoes

MAKES: 1 serving
GLUTEN FREE*, VEGETARIAN

Start your day in a different way! This savory toast is loaded with flavor to help keep you satisfied until snack time.

1 slice (1½ ounces) whole grain bread^{GF}
½ teaspoon Pesto Sauce (page 186) or store bought pesto sauce
1 tablespoon whole milk ricotta cheese
1 tablespoon chopped walnuts (toasted, if desired)
4 (1 ounce) cherry tomatoes, halved or quartered
Kosher salt, to taste
Fresh basil, for garnish, if desired

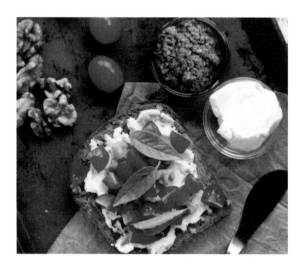

Toast the bread. Spread the pesto on top of the toasted bread, then top with the ricotta cheese. Add the walnut halves and cherry tomatoes. Garnish with salt and fresh basil, if desired.

NUTRITION INFORMATION
PER SERVING: Calories 200; Fat 11g (Sat 2g); Protein 9g; Carb 22g; Fiber 5g; Calcium 61mg; Iron 1.9mg; Sodium 140mg; Folate 22mcg
ALLERGENS: Wheat, Milk, Tree Nuts
* = Gluten Free Option

FERTILITY FOCUS: Whole grains provide fiber, which can help with controlling blood sugar. They also contain folic acid—a B-vitamin necessary for the healthy development of a baby's brain and spinal cord and recommended for all women trying to conceive.

SWEET TOAST

Indulge your sweet tooth with these easy toast recipes that will help keep you satisfied. They provide the nutrients your body needs to power through your long morning, late afternoon, or midnight munchies. And as with our Savory Toasts (page 63), you can make these gluten free by using gluten free bread.

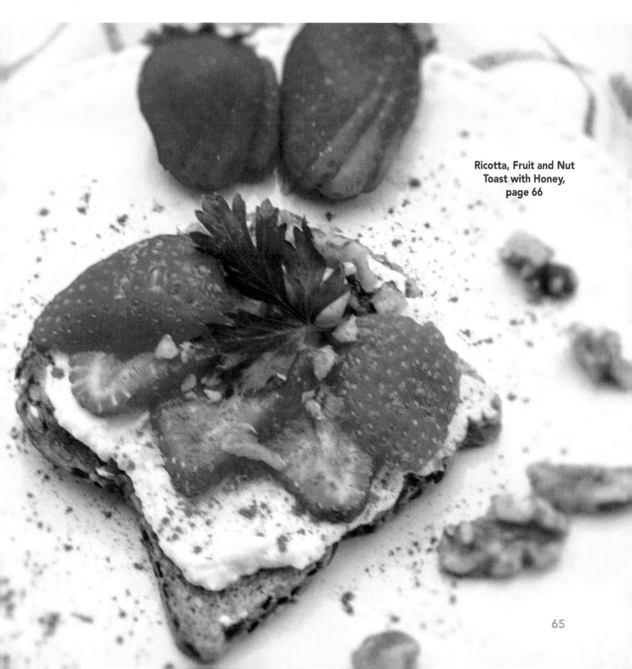

Ricotta, Fruit and Nut Toast with Honey, page 66

Ricotta, Fruit and Nut Toast with Honey

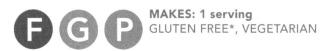 **MAKES: 1 serving**
GLUTEN FREE*, VEGETARIAN

Savory and sweet, this toast provides a balance of flavors to satisfy your morning cravings.

1 slice (1½ ounces) whole grain bread, toasted^{GF}
2 tablespoons whole milk ricotta cheese
½ cup (2 ounces) fresh fruit, sliced (fig, peach, nectarine, strawberries, kiwi)
2 teaspoons nuts, chopped (pistachios, peanuts, walnuts, pecans)
¼ teaspoon honey
⅛ ground cinnamon

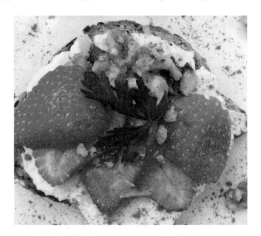

Spread the ricotta cheese evenly over the slice of toasted whole grain bread, then top with fresh fruit, chopped nuts, honey, and a dusting of ground cinnamon.

Variation: If you don't have ricotta, this works well with cottage cheese, too! Simply increase the portion to ¼ cup. Cottage cheese has a bit more sodium than ricotta cheese, but also has more protein.

NUTRITION INFORMATION

PER SERVING: Calories 230; Fat 9g (Sat 3.5g); Protein 11g; Carb 28g; Fiber 5g; Calcium 129mg; Iron 1.7mg; Sodium 200mg; Folate 52mcg
ALLERGENS: Wheat, Milk, Tree Nuts, Peanuts
* = Gluten Free Option

FERTILITY FOCUS: Fresh fruit provides a healthy dose of antioxidants, and nuts supply healthy fat. Put them on a piece of toast, and you've got the perfect combination to nourish your body in minutes. Definitely something you need when you're tight on time, juggling doctors' appointments and life in general!

Peanut Butter and Banana Toast

F **G** **P** **MAKES: 1 serving**
GLUTEN FREE*, VEGAN

Breakfast should be fun! Channel your inner kid and make this peanut butter toast, which has just the right balance of grown-up flavor.

1 tablespoon Natural Peanut
    Butter (page 59) or store
    bought natural peanut butter
1 slice (1½ ounces) whole grain
    bread, toasted^{GF}
1 teaspoon ground flaxseed
½ medium (1½ ounces) banana,
    thinly sliced
1 teaspoon peanuts, chopped
⅛ teaspoon kosher salt, if desired
Pinch ground cinnamon, if desired

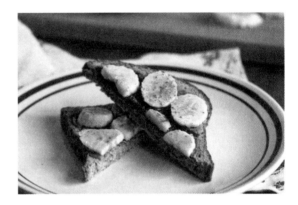

Spread peanut butter on the toasted whole grain bread. Dust the top with ground flax seed and add banana slices. Garnish with chopped peanuts and a dash of salt and/or cinnamon, if desired.

Variation: Other fruits will work here, too. Try blueberries or sliced strawberries for a fun twist!

NUTRITION INFORMATION
PER SERVING: Calories 310; Fat 14g (Sat 2g); Protein 13g; Carb 39g; Fiber 8g; Calcium 66mg; Iron 1.8mg; Sodium 500mg; Folate 64mcg
ALLERGENS: Wheat, Peanuts
* = Gluten Free Option

FERTILITY FOCUS: Our bodies are in constant need of nutrients that can help support continued maintenance and growth. That need only gets bigger when you become pregnant, so use this recipe to help build a foundation of fertility-boosting nutrients to create a truly nourished body.

Sunrise Breakfast Burrito

MAKES: 4 servings, 1 burrito each
GLUTEN FREE*, VEGETARIAN

A hot breakfast (or dinner) burrito that a growling belly will appreciate! This burrito is a filling meal that you can enjoy on the run, filled with protein, vegetables, and whole grains.

1 tablespoon olive oil
½ small onion, chopped (about ⅓ cup
   or 1½ ounces)
1 medium bell pepper (about 1 cup or
   6 ounces)
1 clove garlic, minced
6 large eggs
2 tablespoons whole milk

½ teaspoon ground black pepper
⅛ teaspoon kosher salt
½ cup shredded sharp cheddar cheese
4 warmed 8-inch whole wheat tortillas^{GF}
½ cup No Fail Guacamole (page 116) or
   1 medium avocado, mashed
1 cup Pico de Gallo (page 114) or store
   bought low sodium salsa

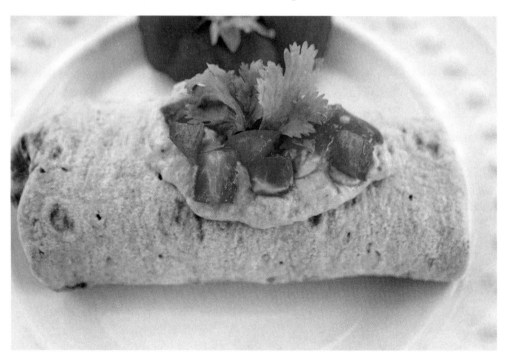

Heat oil in a medium non-stick skillet over medium-high heat. Add chopped onions and peppers. Sauté for 6 to 8 minutes, or until tender. Add garlic and reduce heat to medium, and cook 1 more minute.

Beat eggs, milk, black pepper, and salt in a medium bowl. Add to the skillet and cook, stirring every few seconds until scrambled, about 4 to 5 minutes. Turn burner off and add cheese.

Prepare burrito by layering 2 tablespoons of No Fail Guacamole (or mashed avocado) on the bottom of the tortilla, about 2 inches in from one side. (Note: do not put it directly in the center, or you won't be able to fold the burrito.) Add ¼ portion of the scrambled egg and cheese mixture and top with 2 tablespoons of Pico de Gallo (or store bought salsa).

Fold burrito by taking the two long ends and folding inward. Then, begin rolling burrito until secured. Place on the center of a plate and garnish with the additional 2 tablespoons of Pico de Gallo (or store bought salsa).

Variation: Make it Mediterranean by substituting feta for the cheddar cheese, baby spinach for the salsa, and a tablespoon of goat cheese mixed with sundried tomatoes for the avocado.

Storage: Refrigerate wrapped burritos for up to 3 to 4 days in a sealed container. Freeze for up to 1 month. Reheat burritos by wrapping in a paper towel and microwaving for 90 seconds (or until internal temperature reaches 165°F).

Kitchen Tip: If refrigerating or freezing burritos, allow egg mixture to cool completely before rolling. Omit the avocado and salsa and instead use as a garnish after reheating.

NUTRITION INFORMATION
PER SERVING: Calories 400; Fat 24g (Sat 7g); Protein 19g; Carb 29g; Fiber 7g; Calcium 242mg; Iron 2.6mg; Sodium 710mg; Folate 103mcg
ALLERGENS: Egg, Wheat, Milk
* = Gluten Free Option

FERTILITY FOCUS: Part of creating a fertility-fueling food culture is reminding yourself you can still enjoy the foods you like without deprivation or guilt. This burrito does just that, while also delivering you a hearty dose of fertility friendly vitamin D from the eggs.

Breakfast Flatbread with Salmon and Dill Cream Cheese

MAKES: 2 servings, 1 flatbread each
GLUTEN FREE*

Fish . . . for breakfast? You bet! Fish is a great way to start the day, and canned salmon makes this recipe come together quickly. It's a perfect pre-work breakfast or late afternoon snack!

2 tablespoons Neufchatel cheese
2 teaspoons chopped fresh dill
2 (6-inch) whole wheat pitas, toasted^{GF}
2 teaspoons rinsed capers, chopped
½ cup (1 ounce) thinly sliced red onion
1 cup (4 ounces) thinly sliced cucumber

4 ounces drained, canned wild Alaskan
   salmon, flaked with a fork
Freshly ground black pepper and
   kosher salt, to taste
2 teaspoons fresh lemon juice (optional)

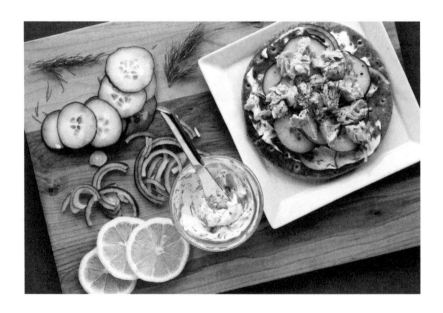

In a small bowl, combine the Neufchatel cheese and dill. Spread mixture evenly on top of each pita, then top each pita with half of the capers, red onion, cucumber, and flaked salmon. Garnish with black pepper and salt. Sprinkle with lemon juice, if desired, and cut into quarters before serving.

Variation: Substitute light canned tuna for the salmon.

Kitchen Tip: Sizes of canned salmon vary. If you purchase a larger can, feel free to add any extra salmon to your flatbread. Or if you have more than you need, remove any extra from the can and store in a labeled and dated reusable container in the refrigerator.

NUTRITION INFORMATION
PER SERVING: Calories 300; Fat 11g (Sat 4g); Protein 21g; Carb 32g; Fiber 6g; Calcium 107mg; Iron 1.8mg; Sodium 610mg; Folate 74mcg
ALLERGENS: Milk, Wheat, Fish
* = Gluten Free Option

FERTILITY FOCUS: Salmon is an amazingly nutritious fish, loaded with healthy omega-3s. Try to incorporate 2 to 3 servings of fatty fish (like salmon) into your meals each week. This helps fuel your body with the essential fatty acids it needs to create the most fertility-friendly environment possible!

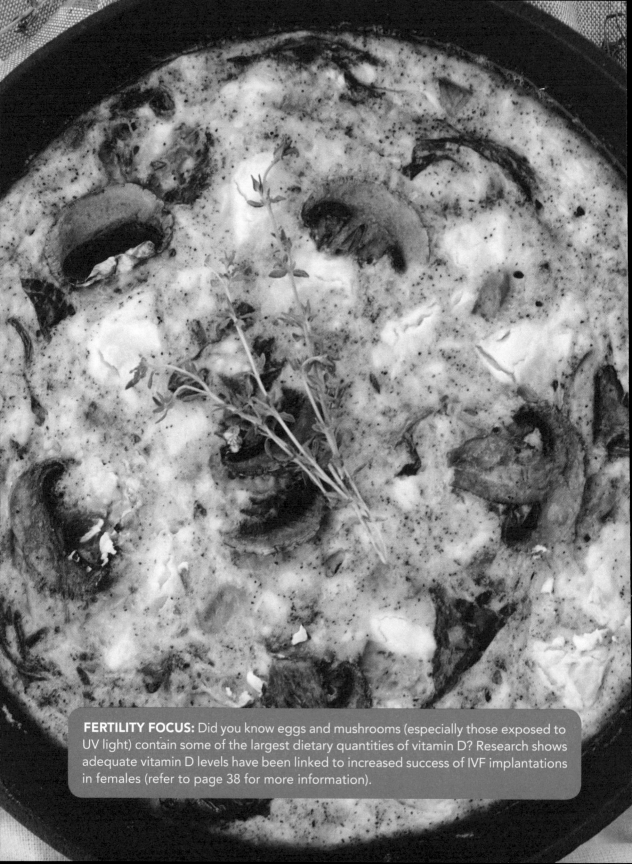

FERTILITY FOCUS: Did you know eggs and mushrooms (especially those exposed to UV light) contain some of the largest dietary quantities of vitamin D? Research shows adequate vitamin D levels have been linked to increased success of IVF implantations in females (refer to page 38 for more information).

Spinach, Mushroom, and Goat Cheese Frittata

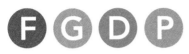

MAKES: 6 Servings, 1 slice each
GLUTEN FREE, VEGETARIAN

The perfect weekend breakfast, weekday dinner, or grab-and-go lunch! This Spinach, Mushroom, and Goat Cheese Frittata will fill you up with its 16+ grams of protein per serving. Pair it with a Whole Wheat Biscuit (page 234) and a bowl of fresh fruit!

⅓ cup whole milk

¼ cup whole milk plain Greek yogurt

6 large eggs, beaten

1 teaspoon ground black pepper

¼ teaspoon kosher salt

2 tablespoons olive oil

½ cup (2 ounces) diced red onion

3 cups (4 ounces) white, button or cremini mushrooms, sliced

3 cloves garlic, minced

2 cups (2 ounces) baby spinach, washed

2 tablespoons fresh thyme, chopped (or ¾ teaspoon dried thyme)

½ cup (2 ounces) crumbled goat cheese

Preheat the oven to 400°F. In a large mixing bowl, whisk together milk and yogurt. Add eggs, black pepper, and salt, and whisk to combine.

Set a 12-inch cast iron skillet over medium heat and add olive oil, swirling to coat the pan. Add onions and mushrooms and cook until onions are soft and mushrooms are golden brown, about 10 minutes. Turn heat to low and stir in garlic, spinach, and thyme, and cook for 2 to 3 more minutes.

Pour the egg mixture into the skillet and sprinkle the top with crumbled goat cheese. Transfer skillet to the preheated oven. Cook for 20 minutes until eggs are set or until a knife inserted in the middle comes out clean. Slice and serve immediately.

Variation: Customize your frittata by adding your favorite herbs, spices, vegetables and cheese.

Storage: Store covered in the refrigerator and enjoy within 2 to 3 days.

Kitchen Tip: The egg mixture can be poured into a 12-cup muffin pan and baked. Spray cups liberally with nonstick cooking spray. Portion cooked veggies into cups, then pour in the egg mixture, filling cups about halfway full. Bake at 350°F for 12 to 15 minutes or until set. Enjoy, or cool completely and freeze. Defrost and enjoy a frittata between an English muffin for a quick "breakfast sandwich" on the run!

NUTRITION INFORMATION

PER SERVING: Calories 170; Fat 13g (Sat 4.5g); Protein 10g; Carb 5g; Fiber 1g; Calcium 77mg; Iron 1.2mg; Sodium 210mg; Folate 45mcg

ALLERGENS: Milk, Egg

Kimchi Baked Eggs

MAKES: 2 servings, 1 portion each
GLUTEN FREE*, VEGETARIAN

Kimchi is a delicious Korean food made of fermented cabbage, scallions, radish, fish sauce, ginger, garlic, and other seasonings. The flavor is tangy and slightly spicy, and makes for a lovely way to enjoy eggs!

½ cup chopped kimchi
2 large eggs
2 tablespoons whole milk
Freshly cracked black pepper, to taste

2 tablespoons chopped fresh cilantro
2 slices (1½ ounces each) whole grain
   bread, toasted^{GF}

Preheat oven to 375°F and coat two 4-ounce ramekins or small baking dishes with non-stick cooking spray.

Place ¼ cup of the chopped kimchi in the bottom of each ramekin. Crack an egg on top of each kimchi-filled ramekin and top with a tablespoon of milk. Sprinkle with pepper and bake in preheated oven until whites are set and yolks are just firm around the edges, about 12 to 15 minutes (or longer depending on your preferred "doneness").

Garnish with cilantro and serve with toast.

Shopping Tip: Kimchi can be found in the refrigerated section of your grocery store. Natural and specialty grocery stores often carry it. If you can't find it at your store, ask the grocery store staff to help you.

NUTRITION INFORMATION
PER SERVING: Calories 220; Fat 8g (Sat 2.5g); Protein 14g; Carb 25g; Fiber 4g; Calcium 110mg; Iron 2.1mg; Sodium 600mg; Folate 53mcg
ALLERGENS: Egg, Milk, Wheat
* = Gluten Free Option

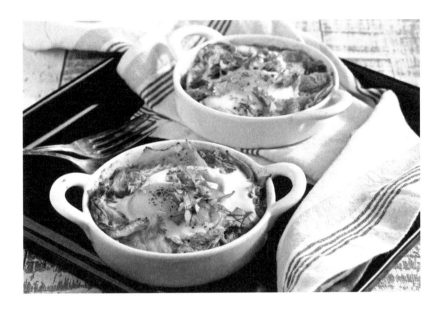

FERTILITY FOCUS: Kimchi offers nutritional benefits similar to other fermented foods. It's rich in good-for-your-gut bacteria known as *lactobacilli*, which are awesome for digestive health. Remember: nurturing yourself for fertility means making sure ALL of you is properly nourished!

Shakshuka (Eggs in Tomato Sauce)

MAKES: 4 servings, ½ cup portion each
GLUTEN FREE, VEGETARIAN

This traditional Israeli breakfast dish is the perfect addition to any brunch. It's a simple meal that tastes wonderful paired with crisp greens, like the Arugula Salad with Apricots and Champagne Vinaigrette (page 147).

1 tablespoon olive oil
½ cup (2 ounces) onion, chopped
1 medium (5 ounces) bell pepper (any color), chopped
2 cloves garlic, minced
½ teaspoon black pepper
¾ teaspoon Italian seasoning
⅛ teaspoon kosher salt
1 can (28 ounces) diced tomatoes, no salt added
4 large eggs
Red pepper flakes (optional garnish)

Place a large nonstick skillet over medium heat. Add olive oil, onion, and bell peppers. Cook 5 to 7 minutes, or until softened. Add the minced garlic, black pepper, Italian seasoning, and kosher salt. Stir and cook for 2 to 3 minutes, then add the tomatoes. Turn heat to medium, cover, and let cook for 5 minutes.

Remove lid and create four small holes in the tomato mixture. Crack an egg into each hole, then cover and cook for an additional 6 minutes, until white is firm and yolk is set but still able to be punctured with a fork. (If you prefer a set egg with a firm yolk, cook for 8 minutes.) Remove from heat and serve with Herb Roasted Potatoes (page 78) or toasted bread.

Kitchen Tip: Crack each egg into a small dish before adding to each hole. This makes it easier to pour and to remove any rogue shell.

NUTRITION INFORMATION

PER SERVING: Calories 170; Fat 9g (Sat 2g); Protein 9g; Carb 15g; Fiber 4g; Calcium 66mg; Iron 1.4mg; Sodium 200mg; Folate 42mcg
ALLERGENS: Egg

FERTILITY FOCUS: The beauty of this dish is that it provides a hefty dose of vegetables first thing in the morning! Plus, shakshuka is made with canned tomatoes, which are a great source of the powerful antioxidant lycopene, known to be a fertility-fueling food.

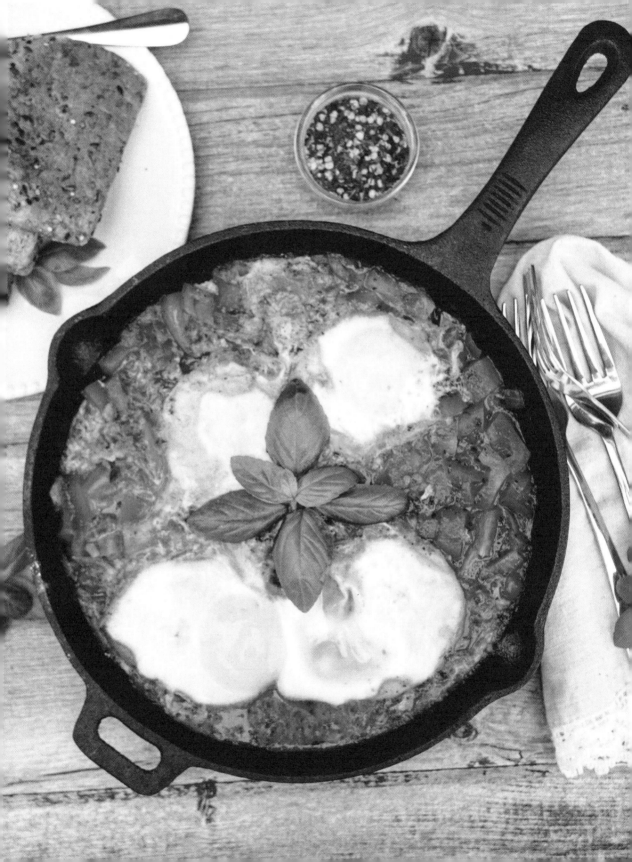

Herb Roasted Potatoes

MAKES: 5 servings, ½ cup each
GLUTEN FREE, VEGAN

Wake up to the delicious smell of fresh herbs and potatoes! These potatoes aren't just for breakfast, either—pair them with the Lemon Parsley Marinated Chicken (page 194) for a delicious side dish.

2 tablespoons vegetable oil
2 cloves garlic, minced
¼ teaspoon ground black
    pepper
1 rounded tablespoon fresh
    rosemary, chopped
¼ cup (1¼ ounces) red onion,
    diced
1 cup (4 ounces) red, green or
    yellow bell peppers, large dice
1 pound Yukon Gold potatoes,
    scrubbed
¼ teaspoon kosher salt

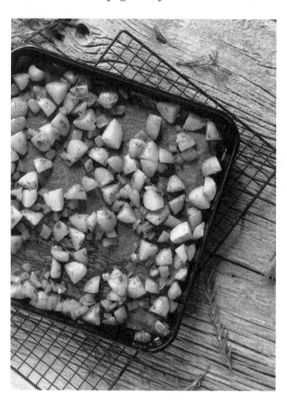

NUTRITION INFORMATION
PER SERVING: Calories 130; Fat 5g (Sat 1g);
Protein 2g; Carb 20g; Fiber 1g; Calcium 74mg;
Iron 1.1mg; Sodium 125mg; Folate 7mcg

Preheat oven to 425°F and place a non-stick, rimmed baking sheet in the oven while it preheats.

In a large mixing bowl, combine the oil, garlic, black pepper, and rosemary. Add the onion and bell peppers. Cut the potatoes into 1-inch cubes (or quarters, if small) and add to the bowl along with the salt. Toss to coat.

Using a potholder or oven mitt, carefully remove the pan from the oven and spread potato mixture out in an even layer onto it. Return pan to the oven and bake in preheated oven for 25 to 30 minutes, stirring twice. Remove and serve warm.

Storage: Allow potatoes to cool completely, then store in a sealed container for up to 2 days in the refrigerator. Note: these taste best when consumed immediately!

Kitchen Tip: Red potatoes can also be used in place of Yukon Golds. Use a sharp knife to cut rosemary, as a dull knife will only bruise and darken it.

FERTILITY FOCUS: It's okay to say yes to the spud! Potatoes fit as a source of vegetables for your fertility-fueling meal plan. Plus, they provide potassium, an electrolyte that helps keep blood pressure in check.

Honey Nut Granola

  MAKES: 4½ cups, 18 servings, ¼ cup each (makes 17.7 ounces)
GLUTEN FREE*, VEGETARIAN

Don't spend money on store-bought granola! Instead, make your own using this recipe. It's delicious, nourishing, and versatile—you'll love it on everything from your smoothie bowl to your yogurt parfait!

¼ cup butter, diced
⅓ cup honey
1 teaspoon ground cinnamon
¼ teaspoon kosher salt
4 cups (2 ounces) rolled old fashioned oats^{GF}
½ cup (2 ounces) nuts of your choice
   (pecans, walnuts, pistachios, etc.),
   roughly chopped
½ cup dried fruit (raisins, cranberries,
   blueberries, cherries, etc.)
2 tablespoons mixed seeds (chia, sunflower,
   pepitas, etc.)

Preheat oven to 300°F and line a large baking sheet with parchment paper.

In a small saucepan, add the butter, honey, cinnamon, and salt. Set over medium-low heat and cook, stirring until butter has melted, about 3 minutes.

In a large bowl, combine the oats and nuts. Pour butter mixture over the oats and nuts and stir until well-coated.

Spread the granola out in even layer on the baking sheet and bake 25 to 30 minutes, or until golden, stirring every 5

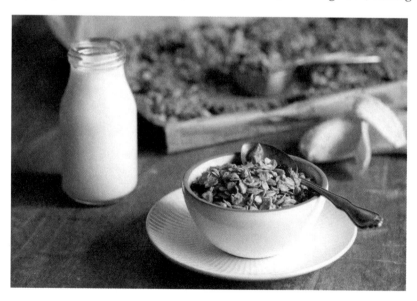

to 10 minutes. Remove from the oven, allowing mixture to cool before mixing in the dried fruit and seeds. Cool completely before storing.

Variation: Substitute maple syrup for the honey, or use half honey and half maple syrup. If you love cinnamon, feel free to add 1 or 2 more teaspoons!

Storage: Granola can be stored in an airtight container for up to 2 weeks at room temperature or up to 3 months in the freezer.

NUTRITION INFORMATION
PER SERVING: Calories 150; Fat 7g (Sat 2g); Protein 3g; Carb 20g; Fiber 2g; Calcium 5mg; Iron 1.0mg; Sodium 55mg; Folate 1mcg
ALLERGENS: Milk, Peanuts, Tree Nuts
* = Gluten Free Option

FERTILITY FOCUS: Granola recipes are often loaded with added sugars, but not this one. At about a half-teaspoon of honey per serving, you're staying within a reasonable limit. This is important as you fuel your body for fertility, because you need to be mindful of your added sugar intake.

PB&J Greek Yogurt Parfaits

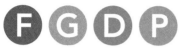

MAKES: 5 servings, 1 parfait each
GLUTEN FREE*, VEGETARIAN

This PB&J Granola Parfait will make any adult feel like a kid again. Your childhood favorites, peanut butter and jelly, unite in a good-for-you yogurt parfait that's loaded with nourishing whole grains, nuts, and berries.

1½ cups rolled old fashioned oats^{GF}
¼ cup pecans or walnuts, chopped
¼ cup peanuts, chopped
¼ teaspoon kosher salt
3 tablespoons All Natural Berry Jam
    (page 57), or store bought alternative
1 tablespoon honey
2 tablespoons Natural Peanut Butter
    (page 59), or store bought alternative
1¼ cup plain whole milk Greek yogurt
1¼ cup fresh or frozen berries

Preheat the oven to 325°F and line a large baking sheet with parchment paper. In a medium bowl, stir together the oats, pecans, peanuts, and salt.

In a 1 cup glass measuring cup or microwave-safe bowl, combine jam, honey and peanut butter. Cover and microwave on medium heat for 1 minute. Remove from the microwave, stir, then pour over the oats and nuts, mixing until everything is evenly coated.

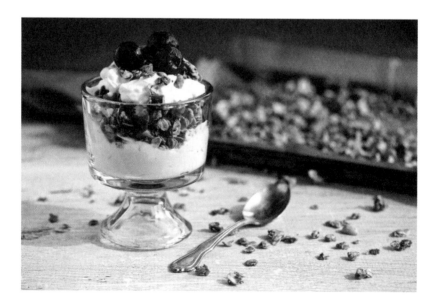

Spread granola out in an even layer onto the prepared baking sheet and bake about 18 minutes, stirring every 5 minutes to prevent over-browning. Remove from the oven and allow to cool slightly.

To serve, distribute half of the Greek yogurt between five serving cups, then layer with half of the granola and half of the berries. Repeat the layers and serve.

Variation: Use other fruit of your choice, such as peaches or bananas.

Storage: Granola can be stored in an airtight container for up to 2 weeks at room temperature or for up to 3 months in the freezer.

NUTRITION INFORMATION

PER SERVING: Calories 350; Fat 20g (Sat 4g); Protein 15g; Carb 33g; Fiber 6g; Calcium 94mg; Iron 1.8mg; Sodium 200mg; Folate 36mcg
ALLERGENS: Peanuts, Milk
* = Gluten Free Option

FERTILITY FOCUS: You can't lose by starting your day with this meal. From antioxidants to vegetarian protein, you'll be fueling your body with the plant-based nutrition it needs to function at its best.

Chocolate Chip Banana Bread

 MAKES: 1 loaf (12 servings of 1 slice each)
GLUTEN FREE*, VEGETARIAN

Banana bread made better! Whole wheat flour and mini chocolate chips make this a snack that everyone will love.

2 ripe medium (6 ounces) bananas,
    peeled
3 tablespoons canola oil
1 large egg
⅓ cup whole milk
1 teaspoon vanilla extract
¼ cup granulated sugar
1 cup lightly scooped white whole
    wheat flour^{GF}

½ cup all-purpose flour^{GF}
½ teaspoon salt
1 teaspoon baking soda
¾ teaspoon baking powder
½ teaspoon ground cinnamon
¼ cup semisweet mini chocolate chips

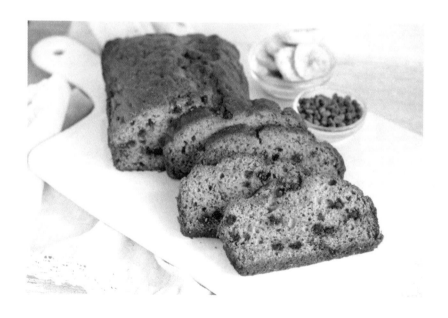

Preheat oven to 350°F and coat a 9 x 5 x 3-inch loaf pan with nonstick cooking spray.

Place bananas in a large bowl and mash with a fork. Add the oil, egg, milk, vanilla extract, and sugar to the bowl and whisk to combine.

In a medium bowl, combine the flours, salt, baking soda, baking powder and cinnamon. Add to the egg mixture and stir until just combined. Stir in the chocolate chips and then pour into the prepared pan. Bake 40-50 minutes, or until a toothpick inserted into the center comes out clean. Let the bread cool in the loaf pan for about 10 minutes before removing and slicing.

Variation: Use a 12-count muffin pan instead. Add ¾ cup whole milk to the wet ingredients during preparation. Scoop ¼ cup batter into each muffin tin and bake for 22 to 24 minutes. Remove when tops become golden and toothpick inserted comes out clean.

Storage: Place in a storage container or zip-top bag and refrigerate for up to 1 week or freeze for up to 2 months.

Kitchen Tip: For naturally sweeter bread, use ripe bananas and cut back on the granulated sugar.

NUTRITION INFORMATION
PER SERVING: Calories 140; Fat 6g (Sat 1g); Protein 3g; Carb 22g; Fiber 2g; Calcium 52mg; Iron 0.9mg; Sodium 300mg; Folate 21mcg
ALLERGENS: Egg, Milk, Wheat
* = Gluten Free Option

FERTILITY FOCUS: Everyone loves a sweet treat, and we're no exception. This quick bread satisfies without the exorbitant amount of added sugars found in many other quick bread recipes. The secret? Really ripe bananas!

Flax Oatmeal Bake with Peaches

 MAKES: 8 servings, 2 x 2-inch piece
GLUTEN FREE*, VEGETARIAN

Ready for an oat recipe that you don't have to make nightly? Make this baked oatmeal once and enjoy it all week long.

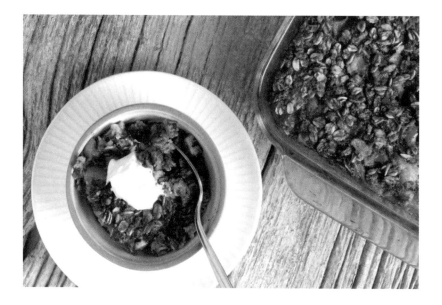

2 cups rolled old fashioned rolled oats^{GF}
½ cup flaxseed meal
¼ teaspoon kosher salt
1¼ teaspoons baking soda
1 teaspoon ground cinnamon
2 (15-ounce) cans (2¾ cups, 18½ ounces) drained and diced canned peaches

½ cup unsweetened applesauce
1 large egg, lightly beaten
2 tablespoons butter, melted
¼ cup light brown sugar, packed
1 teaspoon pure vanilla extract
½ cup whole milk
½ cup chopped walnuts (or pecans, pistachios, or alternative nut)

Preheat oven to 375°F and coat an 8 x 8-inch glass baking pan with cooking spray.

In a medium bowl, combine oats, flaxseed meal, salt, baking soda, and cinnamon. Set aside.

In a larger bowl, combine diced peaches, applesauce, egg, melted butter, brown sugar, vanilla extract, and milk. Pour dry ingredients into wet and stir to combine. Stir in the chopped walnuts. Pour mixture into prepared baking pan and bake for 40-50 minutes, or until set (slightly firm to the touch in the center) and top is lightly browned.

Remove pan from the oven and cool on a wire rack for 10 minutes before serving.

Variation: Substitute unsweetened canned apples or pears in place of peaches.

Storage: Refrigerate in an airtight container for up to 5 days.

NUTRITION INFORMATION
PER SERVING: Calories 240; Fat 12g (Sat 3g); Protein 6g; Carb 30g; Fiber 5g; Calcium 58mg; Iron 1.8mg; Sodium 290mg; Folate 11mcg
ALLERGENS: Egg, Milk, Tree Nuts
* = Gluten Free Option

FERTILITY FOCUS: Whole grains, healthy fats, and fruit make this an excellent fertility fueling combo. Plus, you get an extra dose of protein, making it a great way to keep your hunger at bay and blood sugar stabilized well into the lunch hour.

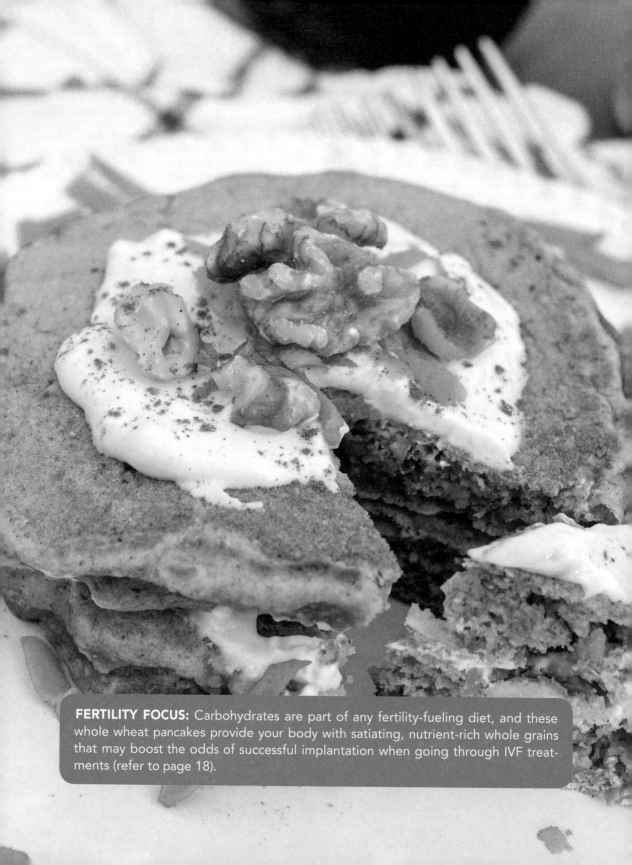

FERTILITY FOCUS: Carbohydrates are part of any fertility-fueling diet, and these whole wheat pancakes provide your body with satiating, nutrient-rich whole grains that may boost the odds of successful implantation when going through IVF treatments (refer to page 18).

Light and Fluffy Whole Wheat Pancakes

MAKES: 8 servings of 2 pancakes each
GLUTEN FREE*, VEGETARIAN

Who doesn't love a delicious, fluffy pancake on a weekend morning? Homemade pancakes are staples in our homes, and they can be in yours, too! We recommend serving these with Greek yogurt or a glass of milk to make it a complete meal.

1½ cups whole milk

2 tablespoons apple cider or white vinegar

1½ cups white whole wheat flour^{GF}

2 tablespoons granulated sugar

1½ teaspoons baking powder

½ teaspoon baking soda

½ teaspoon cinnamon (and up to 1 teaspoon)

⅛ teaspoon salt

1 large egg, lightly beaten

1 tablespoon vegetable oil

1 teaspoon vanilla extract

Fresh fruit (optional garnish)

In a large bowl, combine milk with apple cider vinegar and let sit 10-15 minutes. In a separate bowl, whisk together the flour, sugar, baking powder, baking soda, cinnamon and salt. Set side.

To the bowl with the milk, add the egg, oil, and vanilla extract and mix together. Pour dry ingredients into the wet and whisk until just combined.

Set a nonstick skillet or griddle over medium heat. Once hot, spray with nonstick cooking spray, then drop pancakes onto hot pan using a ¼ cup measuring cup. Cook on the first side until batter begins to bubble, about 2 to 4 minutes, then flip and cook the other side an additional 2 to 3 minutes or until lightly browned. Repeat with the remaining batter.

Serve warm with fresh fruit of your choice or a light drizzle of maple syrup.

Variation: Top with a tablespoon of Chocolate Cinnamon Nut Butter (page 60) and sliced bananas for a flavor-filled breakfast!

Storage: Pancakes can be stored in a zip-top bag in the refrigerator for up to a week, or in the freezer for up to 2 months.

Kitchen Tip: To make these pancakes extra fluffy, we've used the trick of combining milk with vinegar. This helps activate the baking soda and increases the volume of the pancakes.

NUTRITION INFORMATION
PER SERVING: Calories 160; Fat 4.5g (Sat 1g); Protein 5g; Carb 24g; Fiber 3g; Calcium 220mg; Iron 1.1mg; Sodium 160mg; Folate 5mcg
ALLERGENS: Milk, Wheat, Egg
* = Gluten Free Option

Carrot Cake Pancakes

MAKES: 8 servings of 2 pancakes each
GLUTEN FREE*, VEGETARIAN

With these carrot cake pancakes, you'll feel like you're having your cake and eating it, too! Carrots keep these pancakes moist, while the spices are key to making them feel indulgent and satisfying.

4 medium carrots
1¾ cup white whole wheat
    flour ^{GF}
1½ teaspoons baking
    powder
¾ teaspoon baking soda
¼ teaspoon kosher salt
2 teaspoons ground
    cinnamon
½ teaspoon ground
    nutmeg
½ teaspoon ground ginger
2 large eggs
1¾ cup whole milk
2 tablespoons packed
    brown sugar
2 tablespoons vegetable oil
½ cup walnuts, finely
    chopped

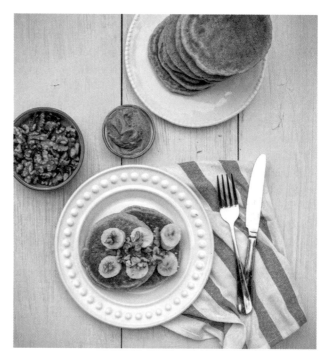

Peel and finely grate the carrots (this should yield about 2 cups). Set aside.

In a large mixing bowl, whisk together the flour, baking powder, baking soda, salt, cinnamon, nutmeg, and ginger.

In a separate mixing bowl, whisk together the eggs, milk, brown sugar, and oil. Stir in the nuts and carrots. Add dry mixture to wet mixture and stir gently until combined.

Heat a nonstick pan or griddle over medium-high heat. Once hot, spray with nonstick cooking spray and drop pancakes onto hot pan using a ¼ cup measuring cup. Cook on until batter begins to bubble, about 2 to 4 minutes, then flip and cook the other side an additional 2 to 3 minutes or until lightly browned. Repeat with the remaining batter.

Top with a little drizzle of pure maple syrup or enjoy plain, right off the stove.

Storage: Pancakes can be stored in a zip-top bag in the refrigerator for up to a week, or in the freezer for up to 2 months.

Kitchen Tip: Keep cooked pancakes warm by placing them on a sheet pan in a 200°F oven.

NUTRITION INFORMATION
PER SERVING: Calories 260; Fat 12g (Sat 2.5g); Protein 8g; Carb 31g; Fiber 5g; Calcium 140mg; Iron 1.6mg; Sodium 340mg; Folate 21mcg
ALLERGENS: Wheat, Egg, Milk, Tree Nuts

* = Gluten Free Option

FERTILITY FOCUS: Carrots add a boost of Vitamin A to this recipe, an important antioxidant that supports eye and skin health and an important vitamin ensuring you are your most nourished self.

Whole Wheat Freezer Waffles

MAKES: 6 servings of 2 waffles each
GLUTEN FREE*, VEGETARIAN

No need to purchase frozen waffles anymore! Instead, these delicious waffles will be your weekday solution. Make one batch, or double the batch so you'll have plenty to enjoy, now or later!

1¾ cup white whole wheat or other
   whole grain flour^GF
2 teaspoons baking powder
½ teaspoon baking soda
½ teaspoon salt
1 teaspoon ground cinnamon
2 large eggs
2 cups whole milk
2 tablespoons melted butter, cooled to
   room temperature (or canola oil)

1 teaspoon vanilla extract
2 tablespoons packed light brown sugar
¼ cup ground flaxseed (optional)
1 cup blueberries or chopped
   strawberries (optional)
1 ripe banana, mashed (optional)
¼ cup hemp seeds (optional)

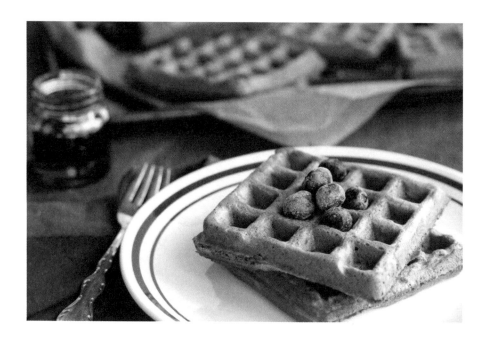

Preheat a waffle iron. In a large mixing bowl, combine the flour, baking powder, baking soda, salt, and cinnamon.

In a medium mixing bowl, whisk together the eggs, milk, butter, vanilla, and brown sugar. Pour wet ingredients into the dry ingredients and stir until just combined; the batter will be slightly lumpy. Gently fold in optional toppings.

Cook waffles following waffle iron manufacturer's instructions. Serve warm and top with fresh fruit, yogurt, or pure maple syrup.

Storage: Allow waffles to cool to room temperature and then place in a zip-top bag and store in the refrigerator for up to a week. Alternatively, place in a zip-top freezer bag, separating the layers of waffles with parchment paper or foil. Label the bag and freeze for up to 2 to 3 months.

Kitchen Tip: To reheat, remove waffles from the freezer and place directly in the toaster or toaster oven.

NUTRITION INFORMATION

PER SERVING: Calories 260; Fat 10g (Sat 2.5g); Protein 9g; Carb 35g; Fiber 4g; Calcium 216mg; Iron 1.7mg; Sodium 520mg; Folate 20mcg

ALLERGENS: Wheat, Egg, Milk

* = Gluten Free Option

FERTILITY FOCUS: Read the labels on some frozen foods, and you may end up more confused than anything else. Preservatives are often added to extend the shelf life of foods, some of which are fine, but others…we're not so sure. Err on the side of caution and, if time permits, whip this up instead!

Toasted Coconut Waffles

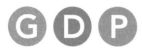

MAKES: 6 servings of 2 waffles each
GLUTEN FREE*, VEGETARIAN

Transport yourself to the tropics with these coconut- and vanilla-infused waffles. No need for syrup here; just a diced mango on top is all you'll need!

2 cups white whole wheat flour^{GF}
1½ teaspoon baking powder
¾ teaspoon baking soda
¼ teaspoon salt
1 teaspoon ground cinnamon
¼ cup ground flax seed
2 large eggs
2 cups whole milk

1 tablespoon packed light brown sugar
2 tablespoons melted butter (or canola oil)
1 tablespoon pure vanilla extract
½ cup unsweetened flaked coconut, toasted
1 cup diced mango (about 1 mango)

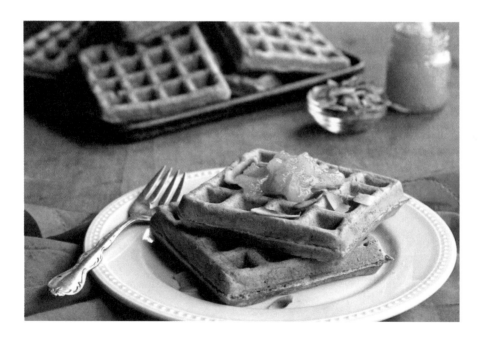

Preheat a waffle iron. In a large mixing bowl, combine flour, baking powder, baking soda, salt, cinnamon, and flax seed.

In a medium mixing bowl, whisk together eggs, milk, brown sugar, butter (or oil), and vanilla. Pour wet ingredients into the dry ingredients and stir until just combined. Note that the batter will be slightly lumpy.

Gently stir in the coconut. Cook waffles following waffle iron manufacturer's instructions. Serve garnished with freshly chopped mango.

Storage: Allow waffles to cool to room temperature, then place in a zip-top bag and store in the refrigerator for up to a week. Alternatively, place in a zip-top freezer bag, separating the layers of waffles with parchment paper or foil. Label the bag and freeze for 2-3 months.

Kitchen Tip: To toast coconut, spread coconut out onto a baking sheet and bake at 325°F for 5 to 8 minutes, or until golden.

NUTRITION INFORMATION
PER SERVING: Calories 360; Fat 15g (Sat 6g); Protein 12g; Carb 47g; Fiber 7g; Calcium 203mg; Iron 2.3mg; Sodium 440mg; Folate 53mcg
ALLERGENS: Wheat, Egg, Tree Nuts, Milk
* = Gluten Free Option

FERTILITY FOCUS: Think you can't eat your favorite foods just because you're struggling with infertility? Not so! These waffles fit the fertility-friendly way of eating because they're made with whole grains and flax seed and only a hint of brown sugar.

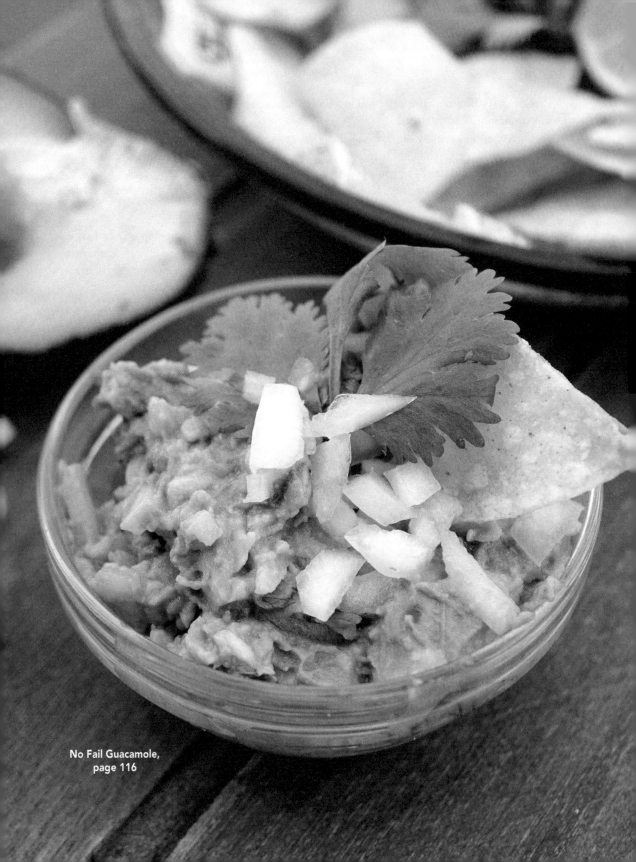

No Fail Guacamole,
page 116

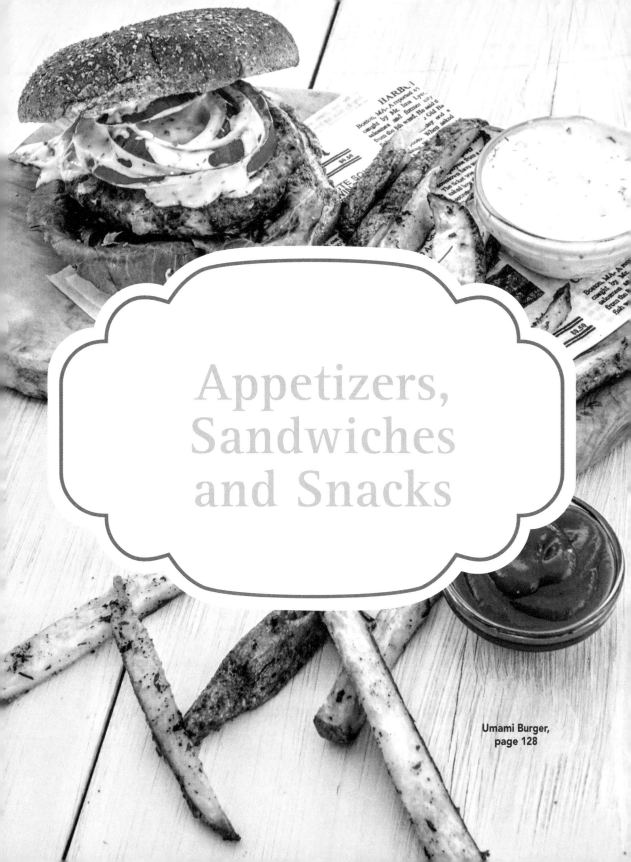

Appetizers, Sandwiches and Snacks

Umami Burger,
page 128

A PPETIZERS ARE MORE THAN just fancy hors d'oeuvres found at dinner parties; they're also excellent ways to fill up your nutrition tank before your main meal. For that reason, we've filled this section with great ideas to help start a meal, *be* a meal, or give something to enjoy between meals.

Sandwiches are the perfect vehicle for incorporating more plant-based foods into your diet, and we love them for lunches as well as dinners and snacks. And speaking of snacks, we wholeheartedly believe they belong in a fertility-fueling diet. Nourishing snacks are the perfect accompaniment to meals, helping to fill in any nutritional gaps.

To help you power through your day, we've come up with a list of some of our staple snacks. Though this list is not exhaustive, we hope it provides some quick fix snack ideas to carry you over until you can whip up that Grecian Grain Bowl (page 208) for dinner!

STAPLE FOOD	SIMPLE FERTILITY FUEL SWAP
Popcorn	Mix plain popcorn with Crunchy Ranch Chickpeas (page 135) and a tablespoon of Sweet and Spicy Peanuts (page 132) to create a savory snack mix.
Edamame	Microwave frozen edamame pods and sprinkle with a dash of kosher salt for a protein packed snack!
Sliced Apples	Core and slice apple into thin strips, then layer with Greek yogurt blended with Natural Peanut Butter (page 59) and top with Spiced Almonds with Chocolate Drizzle (page 134).
Sliced Banana	Top sliced bananas with a little swipe of Natural Peanut Butter (page 59) and sprinkle of cinnamon and chopped nuts.
Whole Grain Crackers	Top with Garlic Hummus (page 103), shredded carrot, and pumpkin seeds.
Whole Fat Greek Yogurt	Layer with fresh or frozen fruit and some Honey Nut Granola (page 80).
Whole Grain Cereal	Enjoy with whole milk and fruit of your choice.

Sliced Cucumbers with Herbed Goat Cheese

 MAKES: 8 servings, 3 slices each
GLUTEN FREE, VEGETARIAN, VEGAN*

Gourmet appetizers are simpler than you might think! These delicious cucumber bites are the perfect way to impress your guests.

1 large (about 8 inches long) cucumber, sliced into ¼-inch circles
2 ounces herbed goat cheese^{VG}
¼ cup sun dried tomatoes, chopped (about 6)
¼ cup fresh basil, sliced
1 tablespoon balsamic vinegar (optional)

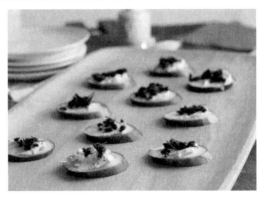

Trim ends of the cucumber and slice into 24 pieces (¼-inch circles). Spread ½ teaspoon of herbed goat cheese on each cucumber slice. Top with sundried tomatoes and garnish with fresh basil.

Variation: Replace the goat cheese with 2 ounces, or ¼ cup plus 2 tablespoons, plain hummus, and omit the tomatoes and basil. To the hummus, add 1 teaspoon ground curry powder. Spread mixture among the tops of the cucumber slices and top with shredded or grated carrot (1 ounce) and a pinch of kosher salt.

NUTRITION INFORMATION
PER SERVING: Calories 0; Fat 2 (Sat 1g); Protein 2g; Carb 2g; Fiber 0g; Calcium 14mg; Iron 0.3mg; Sodium 35mg; Folate 7mcg
ALLERGENS: Milk
* = Vegan Option

FERTILITY FOCUS: Goat cheese is a great alternative to cream cheese, and even provides calcium. Since many of us struggle to get enough calcium, even small amounts are important. Why? Because calcium is essential to maintaining the acid/base balance within the body, while also supporting bone health and muscle/nerve function.

Berry Basil Bruschetta with Parmesan Cheese

MAKES: 8 servings, 2 slices each
GLUTEN FREE*, VEGETARIAN, VEGAN*

Put a fun twist on classic bruschetta by swapping in berries. This dish is great alone, but also pairs wonderfully as the opener for the 3-Cheese Baked Penne Pasta with Fresh Arugula Salad (page 188).

½ (7½ ounces) whole wheat baguette, sliced thinly on the bias (about 16 slices)^{GF}

1 tablespoon + 1 teaspoon olive oil

¾ cup (3¼ ounces) berries (diced strawberries, whole raspberries or blueberries)

½ cup (2½ ounces) diced tomatoes

½ cup (¼ ounce) basil, thinly sliced

¼ teaspoon kosher salt

⅛ teaspoon freshly ground black pepper

¼ cup grated Parmesan cheese^{VG}

1 tablespoon balsamic vinegar

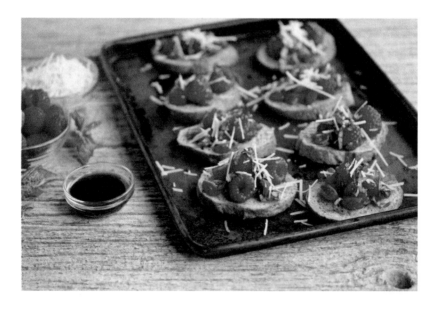

Preheat the oven to 425°F. Arrange the slices of bread on a large baking sheet and brush tops with 1 tablespoon olive oil. Bake for about 5 to 8 minutes, or until lightly toasted.

While bread is toasting, make the bruschetta topping: To a mixing bowl, add the berries, tomatoes, basil, salt, pepper and the remaining teaspoon of olive oil. Mix gently to combine. Cover and refrigerate for 30 minutes to 2 hours to allow flavors to marry.

To serve, portion a rounded tablespoon of bruschetta topping evenly among bread slices, and top with grated Parmesan cheese and balsamic vinegar.

Variation: Goat or feta cheese may be substituted for the Parmesan cheese. A drizzle of honey and fresh lemon zest are also nice finishing touches.

NUTRITION INFORMATION
PER SERVING: Calories 100; Fat 5g (Sat 1g); Protein 4g; Carb 13g; Fiber 1g; Calcium 57mg; Iron 0.8mg; Sodium 230mg; Folate 5mcg
ALLERGENS: Wheat, Milk
* = Gluten Free, Vegan Options

FERTILITY FOCUS: Choosing a diet full of vibrantly colored fruits and vegetables means you're getting plenty of antioxidants that can help fend off those harmful free radicals we discussed in Chapter 3 (page 12). A fertility-friendly diet includes plenty of foods with lots of color that can help prime your body for conception.

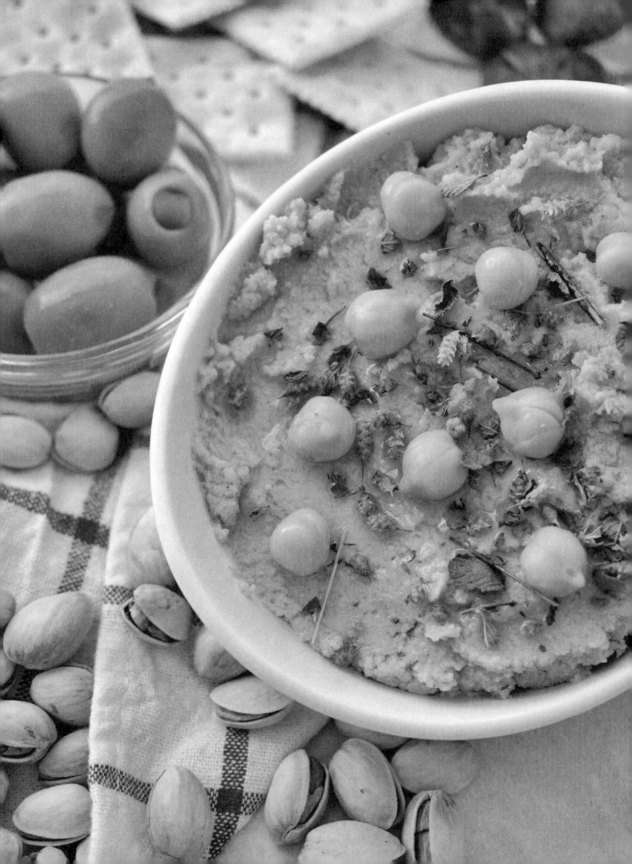

Garlic Hummus

 MAKES: 1¼ cups, 10 servings, 2 tablespoons each
GLUTEN FREE, VEGAN

If you never buy one item again, let it be hummus! This delicious and nutritious dip is easy to prepare, taking only 5 minutes in your blender or food processor. We suggest pre-portioning the hummus and serving as a snack with fresh vegetables or as a spread for the Fast Veggie and Hummus Sandwich (page 117).

1 can (15 ounces) no salt added
  garbanzo beans, rinsed and drained
2 tablespoon tahini paste
¼ cup olive oil
3 tablespoons lemon juice
2 cloves garlic
⅛ teaspoon ground black pepper
¼ teaspoon kosher salt
⅛ teaspoon cayenne pepper (optional)
½ teaspoon ground cumin (optional)

Place all ingredients into the bowl of a food processor or blender, and process for 30 seconds. Remove lid and scrape down sides of processor with a spatula. Process another 1 to 2 minutes, or until smooth.

Variation: To increase the protein and add a flavor twist, mix 2 tablespoons of plain whole milk Greek yogurt into ¼ cup prepared Garlic Hummus. Add ½ teaspoon dried dill, ¼ teaspoon red pepper flakes, and 1 teaspoon of feta cheese.

Storage: Store in an airtight container in the refrigerator and consume within 3 to 5 days.

NUTRITION INFORMATION
PER SERVING: Calories 100; Fat 8g (Sat 1g); Protein 2g; Carb 7g; Fiber 2g; Calcium 17mg; Iron 0.4mg; Sodium 105mg; Folate 14mcg

FERTILITY FOCUS: Plant-based foods can be great, fertility-fueling sources of protein and healthy fats. Females whose diets are higher in plant-based proteins have shown to have higher rates of successful conception than those who consume more meat-based proteins (refer to Chapter 2 for more information).

Jalapeno Beet Hummus

MAKES: 2 cups, 16 Servings, 2 tablespoons each
GLUTEN FREE, VEGAN

Amp up your folate intake with the purple goddess of fertility. If you're not a beet fan yet, trust us, you will be after this!

1 can (15 ounces) no salt added
  garbanzo beans, rinsed and drained
½ cup (about 3 ½ ounces) cooked,
  sliced beets
1½ teaspoons tahini paste
¼ cup water
2 tablespoons balsamic vinegar
½ small (½ ounce) jalapeño with seeds,
  stem removed
2 cloves garlic
½ teaspoon kosher salt

Combine the garbanzo beans, beets, tahini, water, balsamic vinegar, jalapeño, garlic, and salt in the bowl of a food processor (or blender). Process 2 minutes, scraping down sides of processor with spatula periodically. Continue to process until smooth.

Storage: Store in an airtight container in the refrigerator and consume within 3 to 5 days.

Kitchen Tip: To save time, use canned beets, and use any extra beets as toppings for salads or sandwiches.

NUTRITION INFORMATION
PER SERVING: Calories 45; Fat 1g (Sat 0g); Protein 2g; Carb 7g; Fiber 2g; Calcium 14mg; Iron 0.3mg; Sodium 125mg; Folate 14mcg

FERTILITY FOCUS: Beets are an excellent source of folate, a fantastic fertility-fueling nutrient! Folate is an important nutrient that is essential for DNA synthesis and cell division. When trying to form a new life, this nutrient is hands-down a must eat!

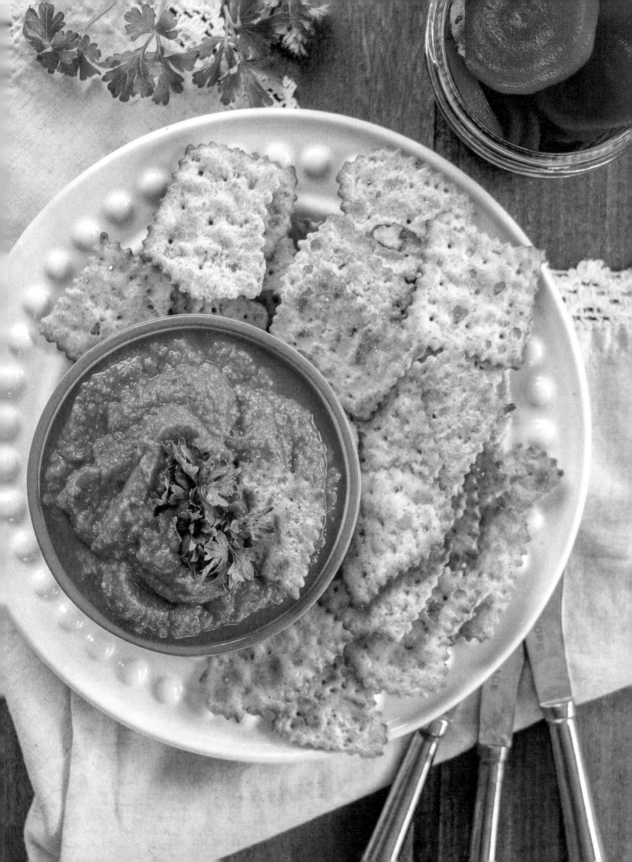

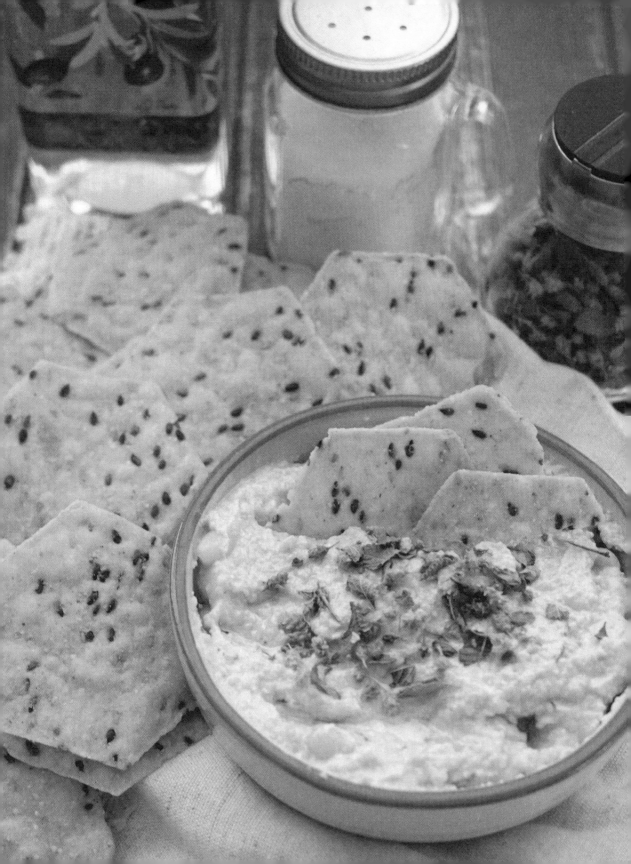

White Bean and Rosemary Spread

MAKES: 1 cup, 8 servings, 2 tablespoons each
GLUTEN FREE, VEGAN

This White Bean and Rosemary Spread uses fresh rosemary and garlic and is simple, yet sophisticated. Plus, it's ready in no time flat! This recipe tastes great on top of the Grecian Grain Bowl (page 208).

1 can (15 ounces) no salt added white navy beans, rinsed and drained
1 teaspoon fresh rosemary, finely chopped
1 tablespoon lemon juice
2 tablespoons olive oil
2 cloves garlic
¼ teaspoon kosher salt

Place beans, rosemary, lemon juice, olive oil, garlic, and salt in the bowl of a food processor. Process 2 to 3 minutes, then remove lid and scrape down sides of the bowl with a spatula. Pulse an additional minute, or until desired texture is reached.

Storage: Store in an airtight container in the refrigerator and consume within 3 to 5 days.

NUTRITION INFORMATION
PER SERVING: Calories 80; Fat 3.5g (Sat 0g); Protein 3g; Carb 9g; Fiber 2g; Calcium 34mg; Iron 0mg; Sodium 150mg; Folate 49mcg

FERTILITY FOCUS: White beans, often referred to as "white navy beans," are a good source of the trace mineral molybdenum. This mineral is important for making and activating many detoxifying enzymes in the body. White beans are also filled with fiber and antioxidants, two things we know are essential to becoming our most fertile selves!

Classic Ranch Dip with Greek Yogurt

 MAKES: 1½ cups, 6 servings, ¼ cup each
GLUTEN FREE, VEGETARIAN

Nothing is more classic than a creamy, delicious ranch dip! Add this to your Umami Burger (page 128) for a flavor packed kick.

Dry Ranch Mix (yield 12 teaspoons)
2 tablespoons dried parsley
1 tablespoon garlic powder
1 tablespoon dried dill
2 teaspoons onion powder
1 teaspoon dried onion flakes
½ teaspoon kosher salt
½ teaspoon ground black pepper

Ranch Dip
1 tablespoon Dry Ranch Mix
1½ cups plain whole milk Greek yogurt
¾ teaspoon red or white wine vinegar

To a small jar, add the dried herbs, spices, salt, and pepper. Mix until combined, then cover with a lid and store in a cool, dark place until ready to use.

To make the dressing, place 2 teaspoons of the Dry Ranch Mix in a medium mixing bowl and add the Greek yogurt and vinegar. Mix thoroughly until combined. Serve immediately.

Storage: Store Dry Ranch Mix in a sealed container in the pantry for up to 3 months for optimum freshness. Refrigerate Ranch Dip in a sealed container and enjoy within 3 days.

NUTRITION INFORMATION
PER SERVING: Calories 50; Fat 2.5g (Sat 1.5g); Protein 5g; Carb 2g; Fiber 0g; Calcium 64mg; Iron 0mg; Sodium 35mg; Folate 0.2mcg
ALLERGENS: Milk

FERTILITY FOCUS: Full-fat dairy may increase odds of conception in women who consume at least 1 to 2 servings as part of their daily diet. Fuel your body with this healthy, nutritious dip while sneaking in another serving of vegetables, too!

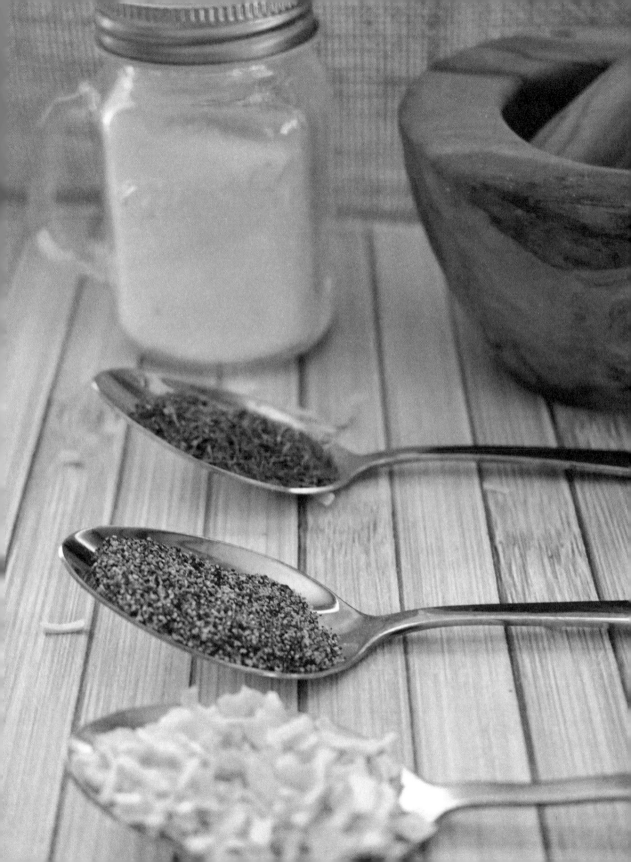

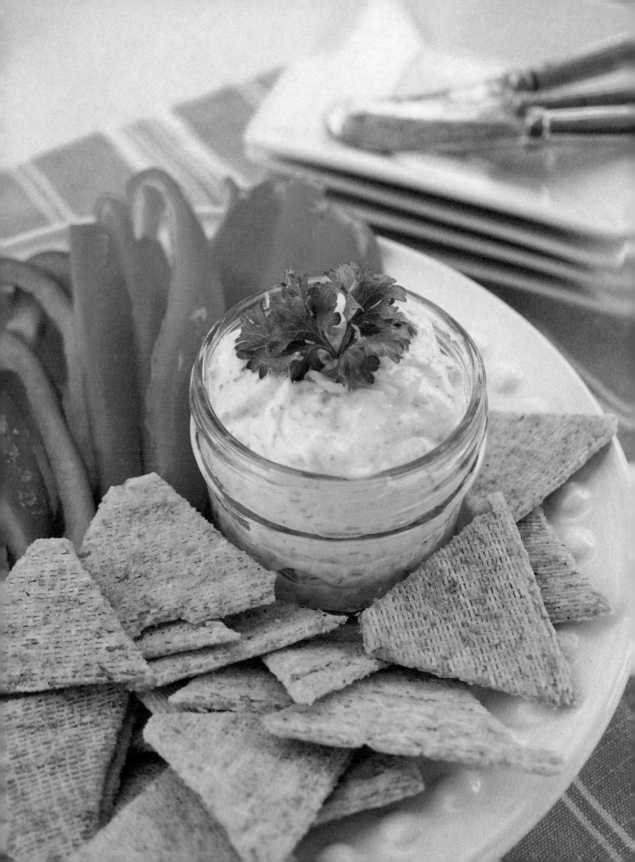

Cool Tzatziki Sauce

MAKES: 1 cup, 8 servings, 2 tablespoons each
GLUTEN FREE, VEGETARIAN

Nothing tastes quite as refreshing as a cool, crisp tzatziki sauce! This is a protein-packed, hydrating sauce filled with pure and simple ingredients. Cool Tzatziki Sauce pairs wonderfully with vegetables for a simple snack or as a spread on the Mediterranean Veggie Burger (page 124).

¼ cup (1 ounce) grated, seeded cucumber
1 cup whole milk plain Greek yogurt
1 clove garlic, grated
1 tablespoon lemon juice
1 teaspoon lemon zest
1 tablespoon fresh dill, finely chopped (or 1 teaspoon dried dill)
¼ teaspoon kosher salt
⅛ teaspoon freshly ground black pepper

Set a mesh strainer over a bowl and add the grated cucumber to the strainer. Move bowl and strainer to the refrigerator and let sit 30 minutes to allow water to drain.

While cucumber is draining, mix Greek yogurt, garlic, lemon juice, lemon zest, dill, salt and pepper in a medium mixing bowl.

Remove drained cucumber from the refrigerator and blot dry with clean paper towels. Add cucumber to the yogurt mixture and stir until combined. Cover and refrigerate for at least 2 hours before enjoying.

Storage: Store in the refrigerator in an airtight container and enjoy within 5 days.

Kitchen Tip: Seed cucumber by slicing cucumber in half. Using a teaspoon, firmly press edge down on the inside of the cucumber to hollow and scrape out seeds.

NUTRITION INFORMATION
PER SERVING: Calories 25; Fat 1g (Sat 1g); Protein 3g; Carb 2g; Fiber 0g; Calcium 36mg; Iron 0.1mg; Sodium 70mg; Folate 11mcg
ALLERGENS: Milk

FERTILITY FOCUS: Store-bought sauces are often loaded with preservatives and other ingredients that may not be "fertility friendly." By making your own, you'll be certain that what you're eating is nutritious and good for you, too!

Oven Baked Tortilla Chips

MAKES: 4 dozen chips, 4 servings, 12 chips each
GLUTEN FREE, VEGAN

We love the crunchy texture of a tortilla chip, don't you? As dietitians, we prefer using carrots and cucumbers as the perfect accompaniment to dips and spreads; that said, we recognize there's no replacement for a delicious chip and dip combo. Pair these with our No Fail Guacamole (page 116) and Pico De Gallo (page 114) for an afternoon appetizer spread.

1 tablespoon olive oil
½ teaspoon lime juice
½ teaspoon garlic powder
¼ teaspoon kosher salt
8 (6-inch) corn tortillas

Preheat oven to 425°F. Move oven rack to the middle position.

In a small bowl, mix together the olive oil, lime juice, garlic powder, and salt. Brush both sides of the tortillas with seasoning. Stack tortillas and cut in half, then cut each half into thirds, to create 6 chips per tortilla.

Place chips on two large baking sheets and bake for 4 to 6 minutes. Turn chips and bake an additional 4 to 5 minutes. Chips should be golden and crisp. Watch the oven temperature; chips cook quickly!

Variation: Feel free to jazz up the seasoning if you prefer a zestier chip by using a blend of ground cumin, chipotle, and cayenne pepper.

Storage: Store in a zip-top bag for up to 2 days for optimum freshness.

NUTRITION INFORMATION
PER SERVING: Calories 140; Fat 5g (Sat 0g); Protein 2g; Carb 22g; Fiber 3g; Calcium 0.6mg; Iron 0mg; Sodium 85mg; Folate 0.3mcg

FERTILITY FOCUS: We promised you all your favorite foods can still fit your fertility diet, and that includes delicious tortilla chips! By making your own, you can control the added fat and sodium while avoiding unnecessary preservatives, three things you need to be mindful of when it comes to a fertility-fueling diet.

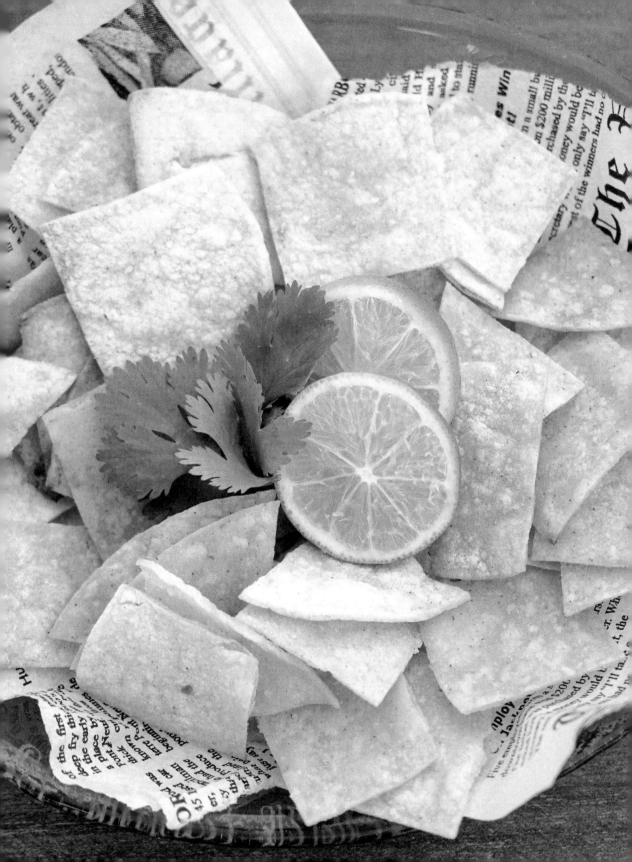

Pico De Gallo

 MAKES: 2¼ cups, 9 servings of ¼ cup each
GLUTEN FREE, VEGAN

Bring the joy of chips and salsa from your favorite Mexican restaurant to your own home! This simple DIY Pico De Gallo is flavorful, refreshing and packed with fertility fueling foods. The beauty of this recipe is that it's literally one of the easiest recipes in this book! Use it as a zesty topping for your Tex Mex Burrito Bowls (page 210).

3 medium (12 ounces) tomatoes, diced
2 cloves garlic, minced
½ small (1½ ounces) red onion, diced
½ cup (2 ounces) cilantro, chopped
1 small (1 ounce) jalapenos, seeded and minced
1 teaspoon fresh lime juice
¼ teaspoon kosher salt

Place all ingredients in a large bowl and mix well. Cover and refrigerate until ready to serve.

Storage: Refrigerate in a sealed container and enjoy within 3 days.

NUTRITION INFORMATION
PER SERVING: Calories 10; Fat 0g (Sat 0g); Protein 1g; Carb 2g; Fiber 1g; Calcium 9mg; Iron 0.2mg; Sodium 70mg; Folate 8mg

FERTILITY FOCUS: We've said it before, we'll say it again: tomatoes are a *great* way to get more lycopene. Lycopene is a powerful antioxidant that helps rid your body of those free radicals which can inhibit both male and female fertility.

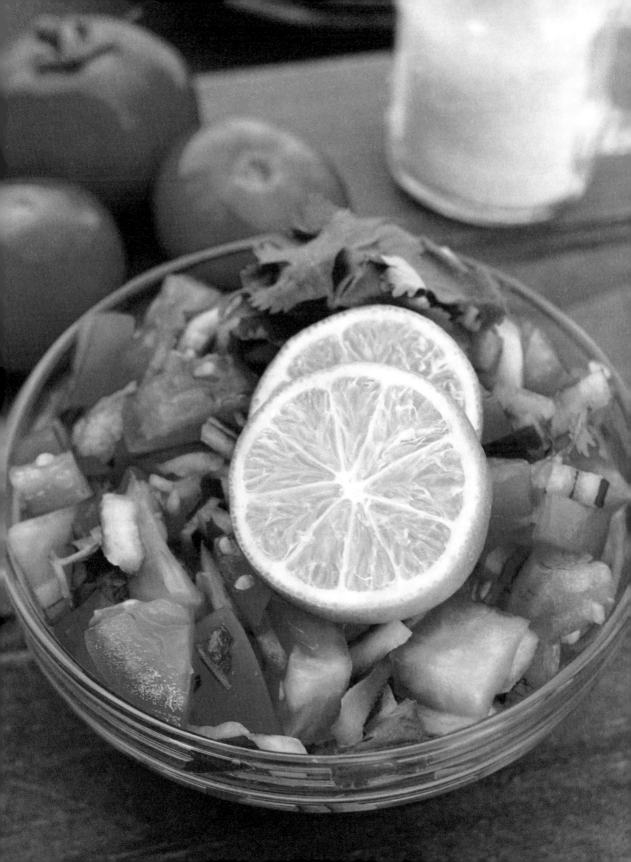

No Fail Guacamole

MAKES: 4 servings of 2 tablespoons each
GLUTEN FREE, VEGAN

This guacamole is simple to make and only requires a few ingredients. Adjust the heat to your preference by removing the seeds and white membrane of the jalapeño for a less spicy version, or leave them in for some kick. We recommend topping Protein Packed Freezer Burritos (page 212) with a fresh batch!

1 medium (5 ounces) avocado, peeled
   and seeded
2 tablespoons minced white onion
1 garlic clove, minced
1 tablespoon fresh lime juice
¼ cup chopped, fresh cilantro
1 tablespoon chopped jalapeno
¼ teaspoon kosher salt

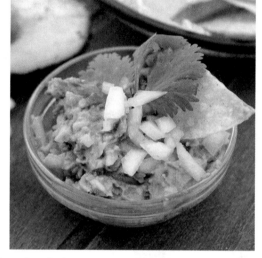

NUTRITION INFORMATION
PER SERVING: Calories 50; Fat 4g (Sat 0.5g); Protein 1g; Carb 4g; Fiber 2g; Calcium 8mg; Iron 0.2mg; Sodium 125mg; Folate 27mcg

Place the avocado flesh in a bowl and mash with a fork or a potato/avocado masher. Add the onion, garlic, lime juice, cilantro, and jalapeño, and stir gently to combine. Season with salt, extra lime juice, or jalapeño seeds to taste.

Variation: Consider adding other mix-ins such as chopped tomatoes, pumpkin seeds, and even chopped kale!

Kitchen Tip: For optimum freshness, make in small batches and consume immediately.

FERTILITY FOCUS: Avocados contain nutritious unsaturated fat, protein, and fiber. Plus, they are a great source of folate, a nutrient that becomes essential once you conceive. Why not prime your body for your ultimate goal by increasing your intake now?

Fast Veggie and Hummus Sandwich

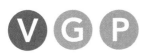

MAKES: 4 servings, 1 sandwich each
GLUTEN FREE*, VEGETARIAN

Your "what's for lunch" dilemma is solved with this simple sandwich, loaded with fresh vegetables, hummus, and feta cheese.

1 teaspoon Dijon mustard
2 tablespoons red wine vinegar
1 clove garlic, minced or grated
2 tablespoons olive oil
Black pepper, to taste
2 cups (2 ounces) baby spinach or
    arugula leaves
8 slices (1½ ounces each) whole wheat
    bread, toasted^{GF}
½ cup Garlic Hummus (page 103) or
    hummus of choice
¼ cup (2 ounces) crumbled feta cheese
1 cup (5 ounces) thinly sliced cucumber
1 cup (4 ounces) sliced tomato

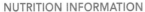

NUTRITION INFORMATION
PER SERVING: Calories 470; Fat 20g (Sat 4g); Protein 19g; Carb 55g; Fiber 8g; Calcium 213mg; Iron 4.3mg; Sodium 730mg; Folate 142mcg
ALLERGENS: Wheat, Milk
* = Gluten Free Option

In a mixing bowl, combine mustard, vinegar, and garlic. Whisk in the olive oil and season with black pepper. Add the spinach (or arugula) and toss to coat.

Toast the bread slices. Lay out the bread slices on a clean surface and spread 1 tablespoon of hummus onto each slice. On half of the slices, add feta, cucumber, spinach, and tomatoes. Top with remaining bread slices, slice in half, and serve.

Variation: Add other favorite vegetables of your choice, including sundried tomatoes, roasted red peppers, or artichoke hearts.

FERTILITY FOCUS: Mayonnaise tastes great, but it's not a food we recommend you consume often. But fear not—other great "spreads" can easily take its place, and hummus just happens to be one of them. Made with chickpeas and healthy, unsaturated fat, this is a spread that's nutritious and fertility friendly.

Broiled Tomato and Sharp Cheddar Grilled Cheese

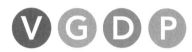

MAKES: 4 servings, 1 slice each
GLUTEN FREE*, VEGETARIAN

Amp up the nutritional value of your grilled cheese by adding delightfully delicious broiled tomatoes. This dish pairs wonderfully with our Lacinato Kale Salad with Peaches and Maple Vinaigrette (page 154).

½ (7½ ounces) whole grain baguette, sliced in half horizontally^{GF}
1 teaspoon + 1 tablespoon olive oil
1 garlic clove
1½ cup (7½ ounces) cherry tomatoes, halved

¼ teaspoon kosher salt
¼ teaspoon fresh ground black pepper
1 cup (4 ounces) shredded sharp cheddar cheese
⅛ teaspoon Italian seasoning

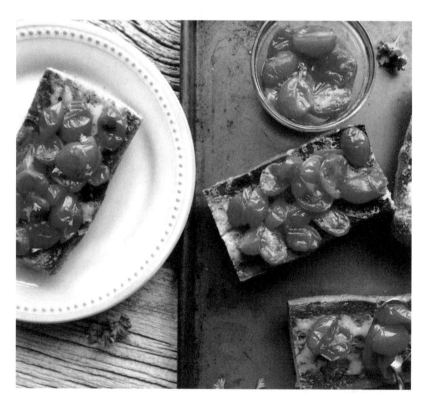

Preheat the broiler. Place the cut on a medium baking sheet. Brush the cut sides of the bread with 1 teaspoon oil. Slice garlic clove in half and rub over cut sides of the baguette. Place in oven and toast 1 to 2 minutes or until lightly browned.

To a medium mixing bowl, add tomatoes, 1 tablespoon olive oil, salt, and black pepper. Spread mixture out onto a small sheet pan lined with foil. Broil for 5 minutes, stirring halfway through. Remove and reserve.

Sprinkle cheese evenly over bread slices, then dust with Italian seasoning. Place in the oven and broil 3 to 4 minutes.

To serve, distribute the broiled tomatoes on top of toasted bread halves, cut as desired.

Storage: Refrigerate in a sealed container and enjoy within 3 days.

NUTRITION INFORMATION
PER SERVING: Calories 270; Fat 15g (Sat 6g); Protein 11g; Carb 25g; Fiber 2g; Calcium 208mg; Iron 1.6mg; Sodium 550mg; Folate 8mcg
ALLERGENS: Wheat, Milk
* = Gluten Free Option

FERTILITY FOCUS: Cooking tomatoes boosts their lycopene content. Can you believe that's all it takes to ensure you're getting more of that stellar antioxidant that's proven to help with fertility?

Open-Faced Cauliflower Grilled Cheese

MAKES: 5 servings, 1 toast each
GLUTEN FREE*, VEGETARIAN

Cheesy, comforting grilled cheese gets a makeover with this Open-Faced Italian Grilled Cheese with Cauliflower Toast. Serve it with a crisp Romaine salad tossed with Italian Vinaigrette (page 161).

1 cauliflower head trimmed of
    leaves and stem, chopped
1 teaspoon garlic powder
½ teaspoon red pepper flakes
½ teaspoon dried oregano
¼ teaspoon dried basil
⅛ teaspoon kosher salt
2 large eggs, lightly beaten
2 tablespoons grated Parmesan
    Romano cheese blend
1 cup whole milk mozzarella
    cheese, divided
¼ cup whole wheat bread crumbs^{GF}
⅔ cup Homemade Marinara (or
    store bought marinara or pizza
    sauce)
Fresh basil, garnish

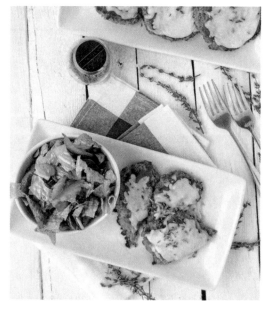

Preheat oven to 450°F. Line a large baking sheet with aluminum foil and spray liberally with nonstick spray. In a food processor, pulse cauliflower in small batches until a rice-like consistency is achieved.

Remove cauliflower from food processor and spread evenly onto prepared baking sheet. Transfer to the oven and cook for 10 to 15 minutes to remove excess moisture. Remove baking sheet from the oven and cool on a wire rack.

In a large mixing bowl, combine garlic powder, red pepper flakes, oregano, basil, salt, eggs, Parmesan Romano cheese, ½ cup mozzarella cheese, and bread crumbs. Mix together. Add cooled cauliflower to the bowl and mix well.

Respray foil lined baking sheet with nonstick spray. Portion and shape mixture into five squares, ⅓-inch thick, and place on prepared baking sheet. Bake at 450°F for 15 minutes. Remove and flip, baking for an additional 12 minutes.

Remove tray from oven and place two large spoonfuls of marinara sauce on each slice of toast. Sprinkle remaining mozzarella cheese over the top.

Bake for an additional 3 to 5 minutes to melt cheese. Remove; allow to cool slightly, then top with fresh basil.

Variation: Customize this recipe by adding your other favorite toppings, such as bell peppers, onions, and fresh cherry tomatoes.

Storage: Place in an airtight container, refrigerate, and enjoy within 4 days.

Kitchen Tip: Use packaged, pre-riced cauliflower to save time. It can be found in the pre-cut vegetable (refrigerated) section of most markets.

NUTRITION INFORMATION
PER SERVING: Calories 260; Fat 14g (Sat 7g); Protein 19g; Carb 14g; Fiber 3g; Calcium 413mg; Iron 1.4mg; Sodium 570mg; Folate 80mcg
ALLERGENS: Wheat, Milk
* = Gluten Free Option

FERTILITY FOCUS: Cauliflower is a cruciferous vegetable that's loaded with powerful phytochemicals. Phytochemicals are compounds naturally present in certain foods that show promise in terms of calming inflammation and preventing many types of cancer.

Chicken Salad Wrap

MAKES: 4 servings, 1 wrap each
GLUTEN FREE*

Packed with protein and filled with plenty of crunch, you'll love the way this is wrap is perfectly nutrient-dense. And we didn't skimp on creaminess, we just lowered the saturated fat by using plain Greek yogurt in place of mayonnaise—the perfect simple swap!

4 tablespoons plain whole milk Greek yogurt
¼ cup (1½ ounces) feta cheese, crumbled
1 clove garlic, minced
2 teaspoons red or white wine vinegar
½ teaspoon celery seed
½ teaspoon black pepper
¼ teaspoon kosher salt

6 ounces boneless, skinless cooked chicken breast, diced
1 can (8 ounces) water chestnuts, drained and finely chopped
⅓ cup (2 ounces) onion, finely diced
2 whole wheat lavash wraps^{GF} (or whole grain tortillas)
2 cups (2 ounces) arugula
8 (¼-inch) tomato slices

Mix the yogurt, feta cheese, garlic, vinegar, celery seed, pepper, and salt together in a large bowl. Add cooked chicken, water chestnuts, and onion to the bowl and stir to combine.

Top each lavash wrap with a ¼ of chicken salad, then add arugula and sliced tomatoes, and roll into a wrap. Slice in half and serve immediately.

Variation: Use rotisserie chicken or Slow Cooker Pulled Chicken (page 196) for the cooked chicken.

Storage: Salad will keep fresh for 2 to 3 days in an airtight container in the refrigerator.

NUTRITION INFORMATION
PER SERVING: Calories 220; Fat 8g (Sat 2.5g); Protein 21g; Carb 31g; Fiber 15g; Calcium 185mg; Iron 2.4mg; Sodium 630mg; Folate 26mcg
ALLERGEN: Milk, Wheat
* = Gluten Free Option

FERTILITY FOCUS: Finding fun ways to add more vegetables to your meals is something we encourage you to do! One easy way to accomplish this is by satisfying your desire for something "crunchy" by utilizing unexpected vegetable ingredients, like we do in this chicken salad with water chestnuts.

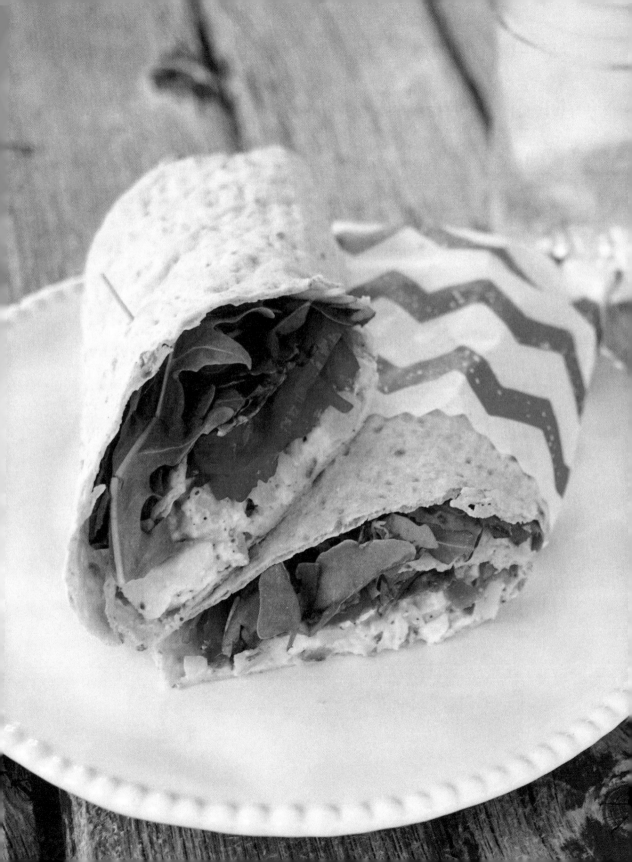

Mediterranean Veggie Burger

MAKES: 8 servings, 1 burger each
GLUTEN FREE*, VEGETARIAN

No need to pay top dollar for a box of veggie burgers anymore! These Mediterranean Veggie Burgers are versatile and taste great, pleasing omnivores and carnivores alike. Enjoy them with Oven Baked French Fries (page 228).

1 can (15 ounces) no salt added cannellini beans, rinsed and drained

½ cup (2 ounces) walnuts or almonds, finely chopped

¼ teaspoon kosher salt

¼ teaspoon freshly ground black pepper

⅓ cup quick oats^{GF}

1 teaspoon + 1 tablespoon olive oil

½ medium (about ⅔ cup or 3 ounces) chopped onion

2 cloves garlic, chopped

1 tablespoon Italian seasoning

1 medium carrot, grated (about 1 cup or 3 ounces)

1 large egg, lightly beaten

¼ cup crumbled feta cheese, plus extra for garnish, if desired

¼ cup whole milk Greek yogurt

5 Kalamata olives, chopped

8 whole wheat hamburger buns^{GF}

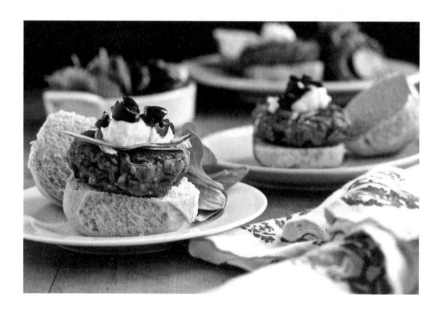

In a large mixing bowl, combine the beans, nuts, salt, pepper, and oats.

Heat 1 teaspoon of olive oil in a skillet set over medium heat. Add onions and cook, stirring frequently, until softened, about 5 minutes. Add the garlic and Italian seasoning and cook until fragrant, about 1 minute. Take the skillet off the heat and stir in the carrots.

Pour mixture into the bowl with the beans and, using a fork or avocado masher, mash and stir the mixture until combined.

Mix in the egg and feta cheese. Divide mixture into eight equal portions and shape into 2½-inch round patties.

Wipe out the pan used to cook the onion and garlic mixture, then set over medium heat. Add half of the remaining olive oil and, once hot, add half of the veggie burgers, cooking 5 minutes on each side. Repeat with the remaining oil and burgers.

Serve burgers on buns and top with a little Greek yogurt, feta cheese, and chopped olives. Or, go the traditional route and top with ketchup and mustard.

Storage: Keep in an airtight container in the fridge and enjoy within 4 days; or, transfer burgers to a freezer-safe zip-top bag and use within 4 months.

NUTRITION INFORMATION

PER SERVING: Calories 280; Fat 13g (Sat 2g); Protein 10g; Carb 35g; Fiber 7g; Calcium 102mg; Iron 2.2mg; Sodium 430mg; Folate 26mcg

ALLERGENS: Tree Nuts, Egg, Milk, Wheat

* = Gluten Free Option

FERTILITY FOCUS: Moving to a plant-based, fertility-friendly way of eating means enjoying more beans! Beans are loaded with soluble fiber—the type of fiber that lowers LDL (bad) cholesterol, which aids in the prevention of heart disease.

Parmesan Portobello Burger with Garlic Spinach

  MAKES: 4 servings, 1 burger each
GLUTEN FREE*, VEGETARIAN, VEGAN*

Mushrooms take the place of meat in this delicious umami-bursting burger! Roast up some Sweet Potatoes (page 223) to serve as the perfect accompaniment.

For the Marinade
¼ cup balsamic vinegar
¼ cup olive oil
1 teaspoon dried oregano leaves
1 clove garlic, smashed
4 (12 ounces) Portobello mushrooms, cleaned, caps, stem and gills removed
¼ teaspoon kosher salt
¼ teaspoon fresh ground black pepper
¼ cup shredded Parmesan cheese[VG]

For the Garlic Spinach
2 teaspoons olive oil
2 tablespoons sliced almonds
1 garlic clove, minced
5 cups (5 ounces) baby spinach

4 whole wheat buns, toasted[GF]

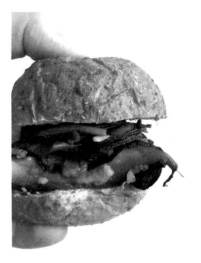

In a large zip-top bag, combine the vinegar, ¼ cup olive oil, oregano, and smashed garlic. Seal bag and shake to combine. Re-open bag and add the cleaned mushroom caps. Re-seal bag and gently shake bag to coat the mushrooms in the marinade. Remove any air from the bag, seal, and marinate for at least 30 minutes (up to 1 hour) in the refrigerator.

When ready to cook, preheat the oven to 425°F and line a baking sheet with foil. Remove mushrooms from the marinade, tapping to remove any excess marinade, and place on the pan gill-side up. Season with salt and black pepper, and bake 10 minutes. Using tongs, flip caps over and bake for an additional 10 minutes. Top each cap with some Parmesan cheese and cook 5 more minutes.

While mushrooms are cooking, prepare the spinach. Heat a large sauté pan over medium heat. Once hot, add 2 teaspoons of olive oil and the almonds and cook, stirring frequently, for 1 minute. Add the garlic and cook an additional minute, stirring constantly. Add the spinach and toss gently, cooking until spinach is just wilted, about 2 to 3 minutes, adjusting heat if necessary. Take off heat and set aside.

To assemble the burgers, place mushroom caps onto bottom halves of the toasted buns. Top mushrooms with spinach mixture and bun tops and enjoy.

Variation: Grill mushrooms by cooking over medium heat for 8 minutes. Flip and cook for an additional 4 to 5 minutes.

Storage: Place cooked mushrooms in a sealed container, refrigerate, and enjoy within 3 days.

Kitchen Tip: To clean the mushrooms, remove stem and, using a spoon, scrape out the gills. Rinse and pat dry.

NUTRITION INFORMATION
PER SERVING: Calories 330; Fat 16g (Sat 3g); Protein 13g; Carb 38g; Fiber 9g; Calcium 252mg; Iron 3.5mg; Sodium 620mg; Folate 116mcg
ALLERGENS: Tree Nuts, Wheat, Milk
* = Gluten Free, Vegan Option

FERTILITY FOCUS: Burgers are a staple in many households, but we recommend honoring "Meatless Monday" by opting for this all-veggie version. Going "veggie" at least once a week can potentially reduce your risk of chronic disease and makes an environmental impact by lowering your carbon footprint!

Umami Burger
(Turkey and Mushroom Burger)

 MAKES: 6 servings, 1 burger each
GLUTEN FREE*

The burger blend is a trendy menu item showing up at some of the best restaurants. But there's no need to pay high prices to enjoy them—you can make them from the comfort of your own home with fertility-fueling foods!

5 ounces white, button, or cremini
    mushrooms, trimmed
2½ ounces onion
2 cloves garlic, minced
2 teaspoons dried oregano
1 teaspoon black pepper
½ teaspoon kosher salt
1 pound lean ground turkey breast
⅓ cup whole wheat breadcrumbs^{GF}
1 large egg
6 whole wheat hamburger buns^{GF}
6 romaine leaves
6 ¼-inch tomato slices
6 small red onion slices
2 tablespoons Tzatziki Sauce
    (page 111, optional)

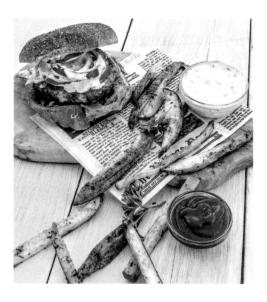

Finely dice mushrooms and onions, and put in a large bowl with the minced garlic, oregano, black pepper, and salt. Stir to combine. Mix in the ground turkey, then fold in the breadcrumbs and egg, mixing gently until incorporated. Form into 6 patties, roughly 4½ ounces each.

To cook on the stove top:
Set a large nonstick skillet over medium heat and spray with cooking spray. Place burger patties on skillet and cook 5 to 7 minutes per side, or until internal temperature reaches 165°F.

To cook in the oven:

Preheat oven to 375°F. Place burger patties on a baking sheet lined with parchment paper and bake for 20 to 25 minutes, flipping halfway through cooking. Remove once internal temperature reaches 165°F.

Serve burgers on whole wheat buns topped with leaf lettuce, tomato, red onion, and sauce of choice (we recommend Tzatziki).

Variation: Use a food processor fitted with a metal blade to pulse mushrooms, onion, garlic and spices. Pulse for 20 seconds. Do not over pulse! Mixture should be thick, not watery.

Storage: Refrigerate cooked patties in a sealed container for up to 4 days, or freeze for up to 6 months.

Kitchen Tip: We recommend using lean ground turkey, usually designated as "93 percent lean" on the label.

NUTRITION INFORMATION
PER SERVING: Calories 270; Fat 9g (Sat 2g); Protein 23g; Carb 31g; Fiber 5g; Calcium 79mg; Iron 2.3mg; Sodium 400mg; Folate 38mcg
ALLERGENS: Wheat, Egg, Milk
* = Gluten Free Option

FERTILITY FOCUS: Umami is a savory taste in food that comes from a compound known as glutamate. Natural glutamate is found in foods like mushrooms, animal proteins, and some grains. These foods can help enhance the flavor of meat dishes to lower the amount of meat needed. Plant-based foods are the most fertility-nourishing foods, making these burger blends a great way to enjoy a satisfying burger while feeding your fertility, too!

Roasted Mixed Nuts

 MAKES: 12 servings of ¼ cup each
GLUTEN FREE, VEGAN

An average serving of store-bought, salted mixed nuts can reach upwards of 25 percent of your daily recommended intake for sodium. That's too much! This recipe shows you just how simple it is to make your own (less salty) version at home.

1 cup (4 ounces) whole unsalted almonds (or alternative shelled nut)
1 cup (4 ounces) whole unsalted walnuts (or alternative shelled nut)
1 cup (4 ounces) whole unsalted cashews (or alternative shelled nut)
2 teaspoons olive oil
½ teaspoon kosher salt

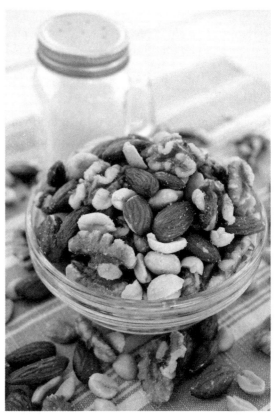

Preheat the oven to 350°F. Line a rimmed baking sheet with parchment paper.

In a medium bowl, combine nuts and olive oil. Add salt and toss to coat. Spread nuts out in an even layer on the prepared baking sheet and roast for 20 minutes, stirring halfway through.

Remove and let cool 10 minutes before eating.

Variation: Mix in ½ teaspoon of your favorite spice blend before roasting.

Storage: Cool and store in a sealed container. Nuts will keep in the pantry for up to 2 weeks.

Kitchen Tip: Buy nuts in bulk bins to save money. Extend their shelf life by storing in the freezer until ready to use.

NUTRITION INFORMATION
PER SERVING: Calories 200; Fat 18g (Sat 2g); Protein 5g; Carb 7g; Fiber 2g; Calcium 44mg; Iron 1.4mg; Sodium 45mg; Folate 22
ALLERGENS: Peanuts, Tree Nuts

FERTILITY FOCUS: Snacks help you get through your day, and when your schedule is crazy with work and doctors' appointments, you need something nourishing. Nuts fit the bill! They're an excellent source of filling fiber and protein and are perfectly portable.

Sweet and Spicy Peanuts

MAKES: 8 servings, ¼ cup each
GLUTEN FREE, VEGAN

These Sweet and Spicy Peanuts make for a satisfying snack. Not only are they packed with a subtle hint of spice from smoked paprika, but they deliver a slight sweetness from a small amount of sugar.

2 cups (8 ounces) whole unsalted
   peanuts
1 teaspoon olive oil (or sesame oil)
½ teaspoon smoked paprika (or
   more if desired)
½ teaspoon granulated sugar
¼ teaspoon kosher salt

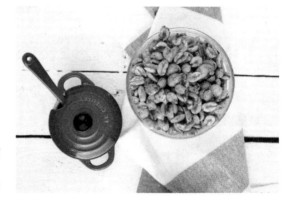

Preheat oven to 325°F. Spray a baking sheet liberally with nonstick spray.

In a medium bowl, combine peanuts, olive oil, smoked paprika, sugar, and salt. With a spatula, mix thoroughly until peanuts are evenly coated.

Spread nuts onto the prepared baking sheet and cook for 20 to 25 minutes, stirring halfway through. Remove and let cool 10 minutes prior to eating.

Storage: Transfer nuts to a sealed container and store in the pantry for up to 2 weeks.

NUTRITION INFORMATION
PER SERVING: Calories 210; Fat 19g (Sat 2.5g); Protein 9g; Carb 6g; Fiber 3g; Calcium 34mg; Iron 1.7mg; Sodium 40mg; Folate 88mcg
ALLERGENS: Peanuts

FERTILITY FOCUS: Peanuts are a great anti-inflammatory food that's filled with phytonutrients. Phytonutrients include antioxidants that can help rid your body of free radicals, which can inhibit your fertility.

Maple Cinnamon Walnuts

MAKES: 10 servings, ¼ cup each
GLUTEN FREE, VEGAN

Step away from the sugar cookies! Why? Because these deliciously sweet Maple Cinnamon Walnuts will crush that craving and then some!

½ teaspoon kosher salt
2 tablespoons maple syrup
1 tablespoon water
¼ teaspoon ground cinnamon
2½ cups (7½ ounces) whole
  unsalted walnuts (or
  alternative nut)

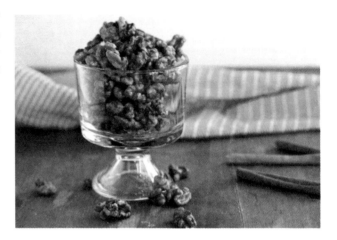

Preheat oven to 300°F and line a baking sheet with parchment paper.

Place the salt, maple syrup, water, and cinnamon in a medium sauce-pot and put over medium heat. Bring to a boil and stir to combine. Add walnuts and stir until well coated.

Spread nuts out onto the prepared baking sheet. Bake 20 minutes, rotating the pan halfway through. Remove and allow them to cool at least 10 minutes before enjoying.

Storage: Transfer nuts to a sealed container and store in the pantry for up to 2 weeks.

NUTRITION INFORMATION
PER SERVING: Calories 170 Fat 16g (Sat 1.5g); Protein 4g; Carb 6g; Fiber 2g; Calcium 29mg; Iron 0.7mg; Sodium 95mg; Folate 25mcg
ALLERGENS: Tree Nuts

FERTILITY FOCUS: Packed with heart-healthy omega-3s, walnuts are a great addition to a fertility-fueling diet. A 1-ounce serving packs in over 4 grams of protein while delivering over 125 mg of potassium, an electrolyte that helps with muscle contraction and keeps the fluids within your body balanced.

Spiced Almonds

MAKES: 12 servings, ¼ cup each
GLUTEN FREE, VEGETARIAN

These roasted almonds are a delightful blend of sweet and savory. Carry them in your bag for a snack, or serve them at your next party.

1 large egg white
1 tablespoon water
⅛ teaspoon cayenne pepper
¾ teaspoon ground cinnamon
2 tablespoons brown sugar
¼ teaspoon kosher salt
3 cups whole unsalted almonds

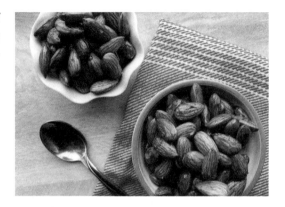

Preheat the oven to 300°F and line a large sheet pan with parchment paper.

In a medium bowl, whisk egg white and water together just until foamy. Add the cayenne, cinnamon, brown sugar, and salt, and whisk to combine. Add the almonds and toss to coat.

Spread the almonds out onto the sheet pan and bake for 30 minutes, stirring every 10 minutes. Remove from the oven and let the nuts cool on the sheet pan.

Storage: Transfer nuts to a sealed container and store in the pantry for up to 2 weeks.

NUTRITION INFORMATION
PER SERVING: Calories 200; Fat 15g (Sat 1g); Protein 7g; Carb 8; Fiber 4g; Calcium 84mg; Iron 1.5mg; Sodium 45mg; Folate 3mcg
ALLERGENS: Tree Nuts, Egg

FERTILITY FOCUS: Crunch and flavor are just what you need for a perfect, satiating snack. We encourage nourishing snacks, but we also believe in moderation. This snack adheres to our idea that sometimes less is more by providing a satisfying snack that fits in the palm of your hand.

Crunchy Ranch Chickpeas

MAKES: 1 cup, 4 servings, ¼ cup each
GLUTEN FREE, VEGAN

Crunchy Ranch Chickpeas are the perfect way to satisfy your salt craving without diving into the vending machine to snag a bag of salty chips. As a bonus, they've got that delicious ranch flavor from the DIY Ranch Mix (page 108).

1 can (15 ounces) no salt added
   chickpeas, drained and rinsed
2 teaspoons olive oil
⅛ teaspoon kosher salt
2 teaspoons Ranch Dry Mix (page 108)

NUTRITION INFORMATION
PER SERVING: Calories 110; Fat 4g (Sat 0g); Protein 5g; Carb 15g; Fiber 4gm; Calcium 29mg; Iron 0.7mg; Sodium 210mg; Folate 26mcg

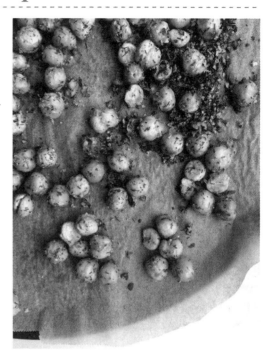

Preheat oven to 400°F and line a rimmed baking sheet with parchment paper.

Use a paper towel to dry chickpeas, removing any loose skins. Add olive oil and chickpeas to a mixing bowl and toss to combine.

Spread the chickpeas out in an even layer onto the prepared baking sheet. Cook 25 minutes, stirring once halfway through. Stir again, then add the ranch mix and carefully toss to combine. Cook 5 more minutes. Remove pan from the oven and let cool slightly before enjoying.

Variation: Try using your favorite spice blends in 1½ teaspoon portions, and adjust as necessary to accommodate your flavor preference!

Storage: Transfer to a sealed container and store in the pantry for up to 2 weeks.

FERTILITY FOCUS: A half-cup serving of chickpeas provides about 1.5 milligrams of iron. That may seem small, but is a great step towards reaching your daily 18 milligram requirement. Iron is an important mineral that helps carry oxygen through our blood to be used for energy—you'll need that for fueling your fertility.

Homemade Granola Bars

MAKES: 15 servings of 1 bar each
GLUTEN FREE*, VEGETARIAN

We know there are literally millions of granola bars available, and some of them are pretty good. But we know you'll love these bars even more, built with nourishing ingredients that you (and everyone else) will enjoy.

1 cup rolled old fashioned oats^{GF}
½ cup brown rice cereal
¼ cup unsalted walnuts, roughly chopped
1 tablespoon butter
¼ cup Natural Peanut Butter (page 59), or store bought natural creamy peanut butter
¼ cup honey

¼ teaspoon salt
½ cup (about 11) dried dates, very finely chopped (or pulsed fine in a food processor)
½ cup dried fruit, very finely chopped (or pulsed fine in a food processor)
2 tablespoons chopped, dark chocolate (optional)

Preheat the oven to 300°F. Spray a 9 x 9-inch baking pan with nonstick cooking spray, then line with parchment paper.

In a large bowl, combine the oats, rice cereal, and nuts.

Heat a small pot over medium heat and add the butter. Once the butter has melted, stir in the peanut butter, honey, salt, dates, and dried fruit. Remove from heat and pour over the oat mixture, stir until everything is evenly coated. Let cool slightly, then fold in the chocolate, if using.

Pour the oat mixture into the prepared pan and spread evenly across the bottom. Using a piece of foil, wax paper, or parchment paper, cover the granola bars and push down evenly on the top to compress the mixture. The firmer the bar, the better it will hold together after it's cooked. Remove foil, wax paper, or parchment, and place in the oven.

Cook for 15 minutes. Remove pan from the oven and set on a rack to cool. Once cooled, transfer the pan to the refrigerator and chill for at least 2 hours. Using the parchment paper, remove from the pan and cut into 15 individual bars.

Variation: Try using an alternative whole grain cereal in place of brown rice cereal, such as puffed amaranth, toasted oat circles, etc.

Storage: Refrigerate in a sealed container for about 1 week, or freeze for up to 2 months.

Kitchen Tip: Chilling the granola bars helps to firm them up to make cutting the bars easier.

NUTRITION INFORMATION
PER SERVING: Calories 130; Fat 6g (Sat 1.5g); Protein 2g; Carb 19g; Fiber 2g; Calcium 8mg; Iron 0.7mg; Sodium 65mg; Folate 7mcg
ALLERGENS: Tree Nuts, Milk, Peanuts
* = Gluten Free Option

FERTILITY FOCUS: Portion size is key when it comes to snacking, and oftentimes store-bought granola bars are bigger than necessary. Their "health halo" also tricks people into thinking that the sweetest, most calorically dense versions are a nutritious snack choice. Not true! Take the guesswork out of portion size by making these "right-sized" granola bars.

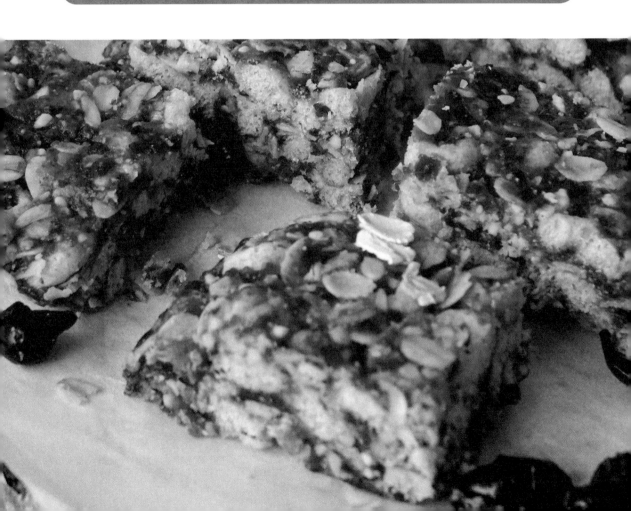

Nutrageous Energy Bites

MAKES: 20 servings of 1 bite each
GLUTEN FREE*, VEGAN

Need a quick bite? These Nutrageous Energy Bites are the perfect way to satisfy your hunger while providing quality nutrition.

2 cups dried dates
1½ cups roasted, unsalted nuts
(peanuts, almonds, cashews, or
a blend)
½ cup Natural Peanut Butter (page 59
or alternative natural creamy nut
butter)
1 cup rolled old fashioned oats^{GF}
¼ teaspoon kosher salt

Place the dates into a 12-cup food processor fitted with the metal blade and process for 2 to 3 minutes. Remove lid and scrape down sides with a spatula. Process for 1 to 2 minutes more, until dates resemble a thick jam.

Add roasted nuts and nut butter to the processor and process for 3 to 5 minutes. Add the oats and salt and process an additional 1 to 2 minutes. Mixture should be coarse and hold shape when formed into a ball.

Using a large tablespoon, shape dough into 20 bite-sized balls and place on a baking sheet. Cover with plastic wrap and refrigerate for at least 30 minutes to firm up before enjoying.

Storage: Refrigerate in a sealed container for about 1 week. Freeze for up to 2 months for optimal freshness.

NUTRITION INFORMATION
PER SERVING: Calories 160; Fat 10g (Sat 1g); Protein 4g; Carb 19g; Fiber 3g; Calcium 21mg; Iron 0.8mg; Sodium 55mg; Folate 16mcg
ALLERGENS: Peanuts, Tree Nuts
* = Gluten Free Option

FERTILITY FOCUS: Focus on fueling your body with wholesome foods that will help you feel better, allowing you to channel that good energy into lowering your overall stress and giving your body a chance to relax.

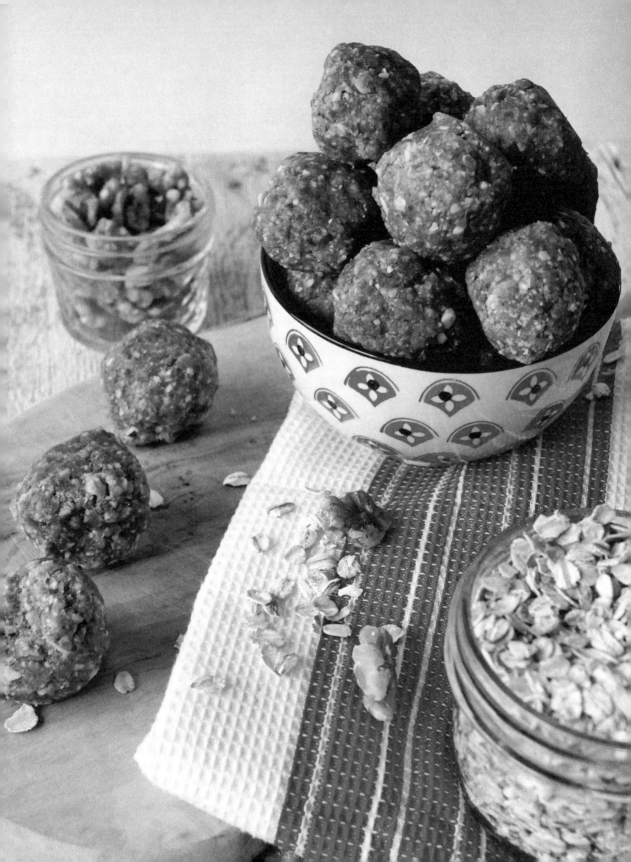

GREEK YOGURT SMOOTHIES

We know it can be hard to think about food and nourishment when trying to manage a multitude of doctors' appointments, let alone balancing work and life; that's why we love these smoothie recipes. They're easy to make and provide the nourishment you need to keep your body running.

FERTILITY FOCUS: Store-bought smoothies can be a great on-the-go choice, but many of them are made with concentrated juices and plenty of sugar. That's not what your body needs. If you have a few minutes and a blender, then you can make these nourishing smoothies that taste great, at a fraction of the price.

Strawberry Banana Smoothie

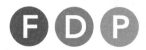

MAKES: 1 serving
GLUTEN FREE, VEGETARIAN

½ cup whole milk plain Greek
   yogurt
¼ cup whole milk
1 tablespoon ground flax seed
½ cup frozen unsweetened
   strawberries (about 5 or 6)
½ medium ripe banana

Place all the ingredients in a blender and puree until smooth. Enjoy immediately.

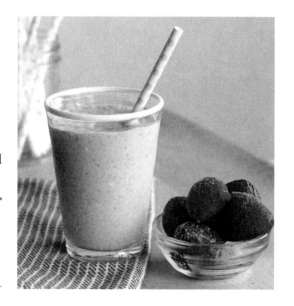

NUTRITION INFORMATION
PER SERVING: Calories 240; Fat 9g (Sat 4g); Protein 15g; Carb 29g; Fiber 5g; Calcium 218mg; Iron 0.9mg; Sodium 65mg; Folate 15mcg
ALLERGENS: Milk

Chocolate Cherry Smoothie

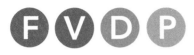

MAKES: 1 serving
GLUTEN FREE, VEGETARIAN

½ cup whole milk plain Greek yogurt
1 tablespoon dark chocolate cocoa
    powder
¼ cup whole milk
½ cup frozen unsweetened cherries
½ medium ripe banana
½ cup packed spinach

Place all the ingredients in a blender and puree until smooth. Enjoy immediately.

Kitchen Tip: Choose naturally sweet cherries, labeled "sweet cherries" on the package, over sour cherries.

NUTRITION INFORMATION
PER SERVING: Calories 250; Fat 7g (Sat 4g); Protein 15g; Carb 37g; Fiber 6g; Calcium 261mg; Iron 2.5mg; Sodium 110mg; Folate 122mcg
ALLERGENS: Milk

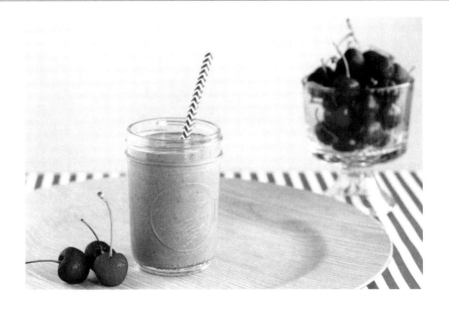

Tropical Fruit Smoothie with Coconut Water

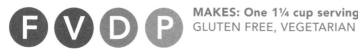

MAKES: One 1¼ cup serving
GLUTEN FREE, VEGETARIAN

½ cup whole milk plain Greek yogurt
¼ cup coconut water
½ cup frozen mango, diced
½ cup frozen pineapple, diced
½ medium ripe banana
¼ cup packed shredded carrot

Place all the ingredients in a blender and puree until smooth. Enjoy.

NUTRITION INFORMATION
PER SERVING: Calories 220; Fat 4.5g (Sat 3g); Protein 11g; Carb 38g; Fiber 3g; Calcium 156mg; Iron 0.5mg; Sodium 50mg; Folate 12mcg
ALLERGENS: Tree Nuts, Milk

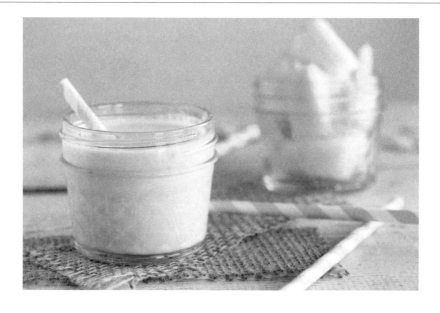

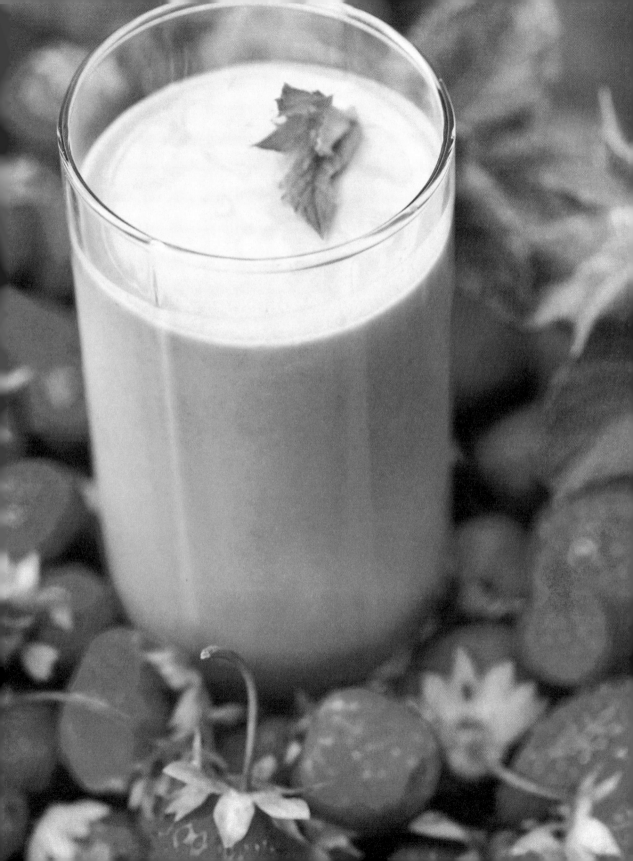

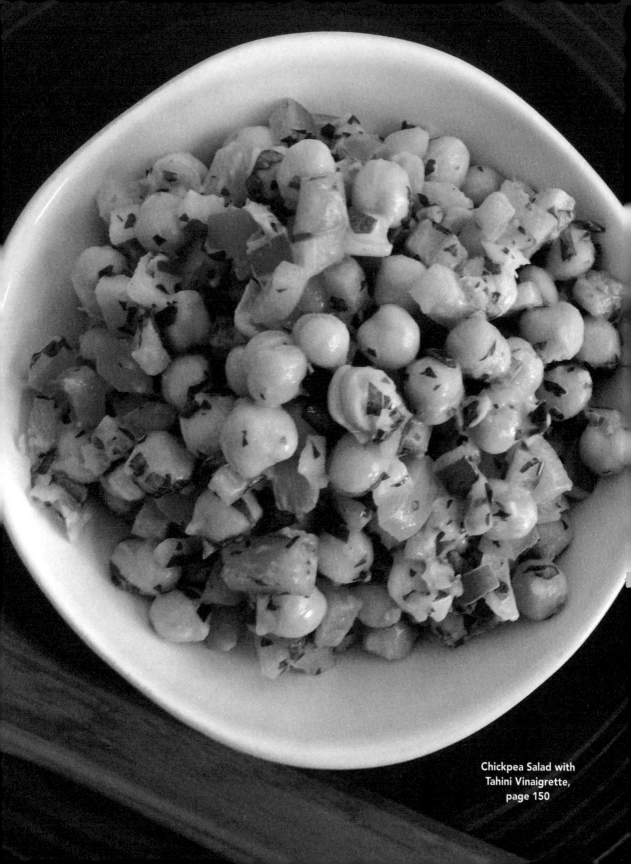

Chickpea Salad with
Tahini Vinaigrette,
page 150

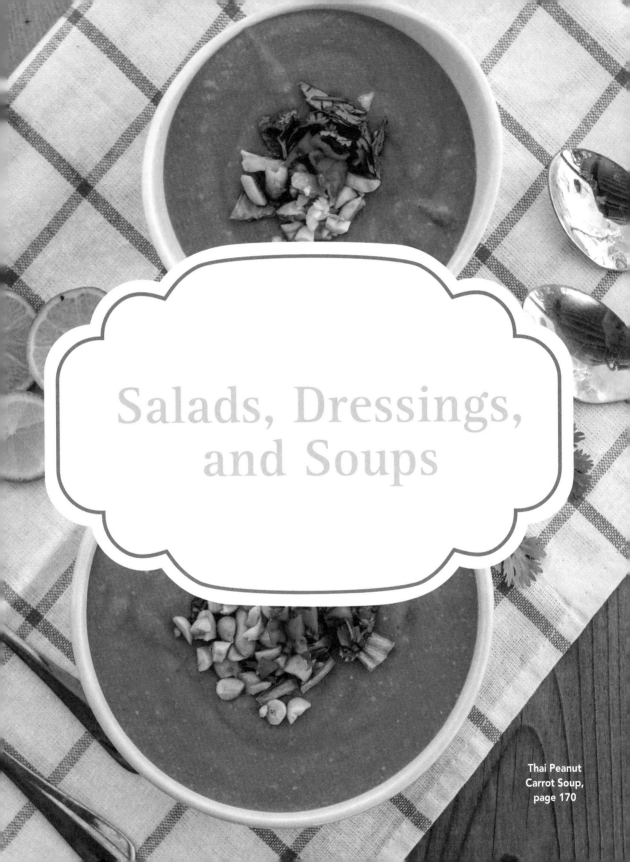

Salads, Dressings, and Soups

Thai Peanut
Carrot Soup,
page 170

D ON'T YOU JUST FEEL better when you give your body fresh, vibrant greens and hearty, plant-forward soups? We do, too! (That's why this section is one of the longest of the book.)

These satisfying soups, delicious salads, and homemade dressings are a great way to fill up on nutrient-dense foods that will nourish your mind, body, and soul—three important things to keep you in great "shape" when struggling with fertility.

If you're tight on time and aren't sure what the best options are when dining out, here are some quick tips to help you make the best, fertility-friendly choices.

DINING OUT: MENU ITEM	FERTILITY FUEL CHOICE
Soup	Opt for a broth or tomato-based, hearty vegetable soup with lean proteins and whole grains. Best choices include: Minestrone, Lentil, Chicken, Tomato, Vegetable, Noodle and Bean Soups.
Salad	Choose a salad with plenty of vegetables, making sure to add a protein (quinoa, beans, grilled chicken, or tofu) and a healthy fat (avocado, nuts or cheese).
Dressings	Vinaigrettes and oil-based dressings are usually your best options. Ask for the dressing on the side and use 1 to 2 tablespoons.

Arugula Salad with Apricots and Champagne Vinaigrette

MAKES: 4 servings, 1 salad each
GLUTEN FREE, VEGETARIAN, VEGAN*

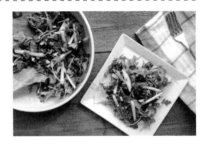

Arugula tastes divine tossed with dried apricots, pistachios, fresh apple, and a subtle champagne vinaigrette! Top this with a little bit of that Slow Cooker Pulled Chicken (page 196) and you've got yourself a satisfying meal.

2 teaspoons Dijon mustard
1 teaspoon honey
1 tablespoon champagne vinegar
2 tablespoons olive oil
⅛ teaspoon dried thyme leaves
4 cups (2 ounces) baby arugula, washed
½ medium (2½ ounces) Fuji apple, cored and julienned
¼ cup (1½ ounces) dried apricots, diced
¼ cup crumbled feta cheese^VG
¼ cup roasted, salted pistachios, roughly chopped

In a small bowl, whisk together the mustard, honey, and vinegar. Pour in the olive oil and whisk until combined. Stir in the dried thyme.

In a large salad or mixing bowl, add the baby arugula, apple, apricots, feta cheese, and pistachios. Pour dressing over the salad and toss to combine. Portion onto plates and enjoy.

Storage: Keep dressing separate if you plan to save a portion for later. Add dressing prior to assembly. Refrigerate undressed for up to 2 days in an airtight container.

Shopping Tip: Champagne vinegar can be found in the condiment aisle at your local market.

Kitchen Tip: Julienne is a type of knife cut that means to finely slice into thin strips. Refer to page 274 to learn about this and other knife cuts.

NUTRITION INFORMATION
PER SERVING: Calories 170; Fat 12g (Sat 2.5g); Protein 4g; Carb 13g; Fiber 2g; Calcium 85mg; Iron 0.9mg; Sodium 190mg; Folate 18mcg
ALLERGENS: Milk, Tree Nuts
* = Vegan Option

FERTILITY FOCUS: Produce plays a crucial role in fertility. Filled with fiber, vitamins, and antioxidants, including a salad a day into your regular eating pattern will provide your body with optimum nutrition to ready yourself for the next stage of your fertility journey.

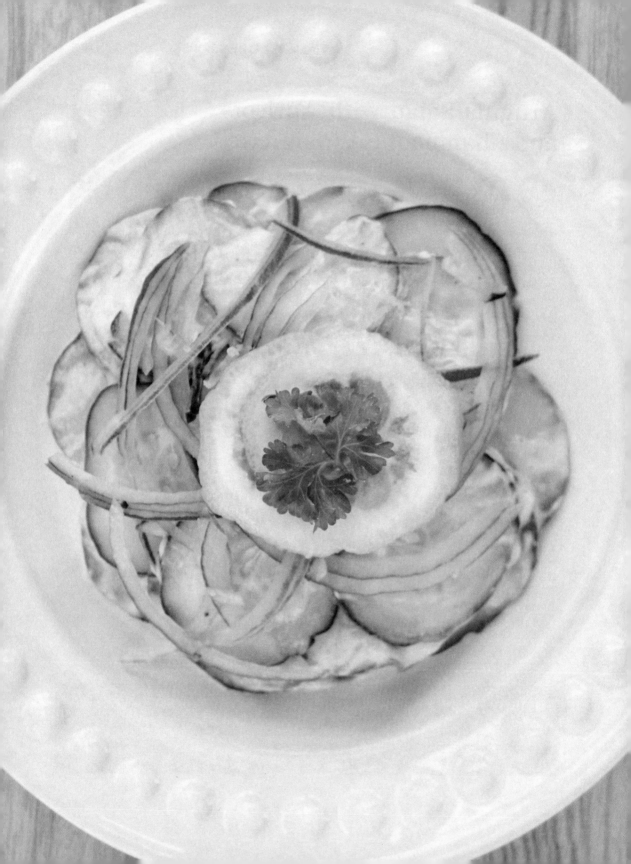

Indian Cucumber Salad with Creamy Yogurt Dressing

 MAKES: 4 servings of ½ cup each
GLUTEN FREE, VEGETARIAN

Everyone likes a creamy side salad. Filled with fresh, crisp cucumbers and tossed with Greek yogurt, this makes the perfect side for the Baked Mediterranean Chicken (page 198).

1 large (about 8 ounces) cucumber, ⅛-inch slices, ends trimmed
¼ teaspoon kosher salt
½ cup plain whole milk Greek yogurt
½ teaspoon garam masala
1 teaspoon lemon juice
½ small (1 ounce) red onion, thinly sliced
½ teaspoon lemon zest

Place sliced cucumbers in a medium bowl and sprinkle with salt. Let sit for 20 minutes for water to drain. Pat cucumbers dry using a paper towel and drain excess water from bowl.

In a separate bowl, mix together the yogurt, garam masala, and lemon juice.

Add the onions to the cucumber bowl and pour the dressing over the top of the salad. Mix together and garnish with lemon zest.

Storage: Refrigerate in sealed container and eat within a day.

Kitchen Tip: Substitute ¼ + ⅛ teaspoon cumin and ⅛ teaspoon allspice for garam masala.

NUTRITION INFORMATION
PER SERVING: Calories 35; Fat 1.5g (Sat 1g); Protein 3g; Carb 4; Fiber 1g; Calcium 46mg; Iron 0.2mg; Sodium 160mg; Folate 12mcg
ALLERGENS: Milk

FERTILITY FOCUS: Just like that Cool Tzatziki Sauce (page 111), this recipe is filled with hydrating cucumbers. Proper hydration is crucial for hormonal balance and general well-being, two essential components of fertility.

Chickpea Salad with Tahini Vinaigrette

MAKES: 4 servings
GLUTEN FREE, VEGETARIAN

A refreshing yet hearty salad made with chickpeas, bell peppers, and parsley, all tossed in a tangy lemon–tahini dressing.

1 clove garlic, minced
1 tablespoon tahini
2 tablespoons fresh lemon juice
1 teaspoon honey
1 tablespoon olive oil
1 tablespoon water
1 can (15 ounces) no salt added
  chickpeas, drained and rinsed

1 red or orange bell pepper, seeded
  and diced (about 1 cup)
1 cup diced red onion (4 ounces)
1 cup (1½ ounces) curly parsley,
  chopped
¼ teaspoon kosher salt
¼ teaspoon black pepper

In the bottom of a mixing bowl, whisk together the garlic, tahini, lemon juice, and honey. Add the olive oil and continue whisking until combined, then add the water. Add the chickpeas, bell pepper, red onion, and parsley, and toss to coat. Season with salt and pepper.

Storage: Keep dressing separate if you plan to save a portion for later. Add dressing prior to eating. Refrigerate for up to 7 days in a sealed container.

NUTRITION INFORMATION
PER SERVING: Calories 180; Fat 7g (Sat 1g); Protein 6g; Carb 24g; Fiber 6g; Calcium 68mg; Iron 2.0mg; Sodium 160mg; Folate 78mcg

FERTILITY FOCUS: Chickpeas are an excellent source of plant-based protein, which provide filling fiber. Studies point to plant based proteins for fertility, showing higher rates of conception with those who consume a predominantly plant-based diet.

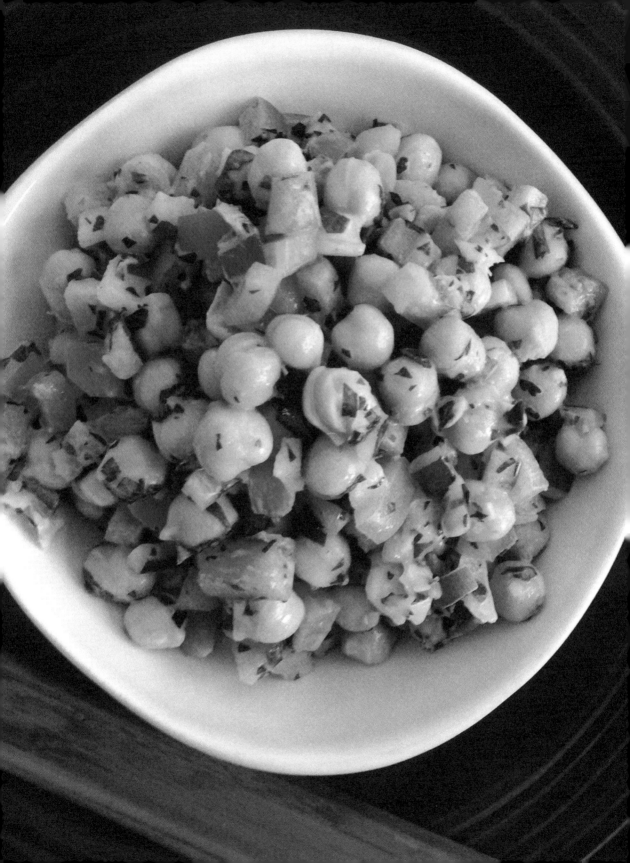

Black Bean Salad with Honey-Lime Vinaigrette

MAKES: 8 servings
GLUTEN FREE, VEGETARIAN

This delightfully healthy veggie-full dish comes together fast, looks beautiful, and tastes great, too!

1 ear of fresh corn, shucked and cleaned (or 1 cup cooked, cooled corn kernels)

1 can (15 ounces) no salt added black beans, rinsed and drained

1 can (15 ounces) no salt added kidney beans, rinsed and drained

1 red or yellow bell pepper, seeded, stemmed and diced

1 green bell pepper, seeded, stemmed and diced

½ medium red onion, peeled and diced

½ cup fresh cilantro leaves, roughly chopped

½ jalapeño, seeded and diced

1 teaspoon Dijon mustard

1 lime, zested and juiced

2 tablespoons honey

⅓ cup olive oil

⅛ teaspoon kosher salt

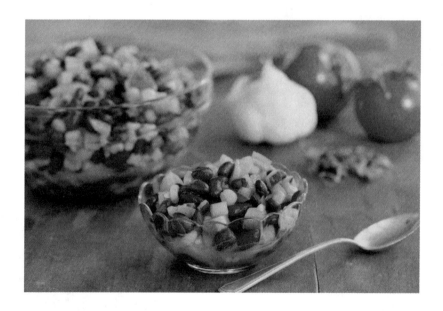

Bring a pot of water to a boil. Add corn and return to a boil. Cook for 5 minutes, then drain and rinse under cold water to stop the cooking process. Pat dry.

When cool enough to touch, cut kernels from the cob and add to a large serving or mixing bowl.

To the same bowl, add the black and kidney beans, bell peppers, onion, cilantro, and jalapeño. Toss to combine.

For the dressing, combine the mustard, lime zest, lime juice, and honey in a small bowl. Whisk in the olive oil.

To serve, pour the dressing over the salad and toss to evenly coat. Cover the bowl with a lid or plastic wrap and refrigerate for at least an hour. Toss again before serving.

Variation: Use 1¾ cups Mexican Black Beans from Scratch (page 242) in place of the black beans.

Storage: Keep dressing separate if you plan to save a portion for later. Add dressing prior to consuming. Refrigerate for up to 5 days in an airtight container.

NUTRITION INFORMATION
PER SERVING: Calories 220; Fat 10g (Sat 1.5g); Protein 7g; Carb 28g; Fiber 8g; Calcium 40mg; Iron 2.0mg; Sodium 180mg; Folate 54mcg

FERTILITY FOCUS: Spice up your lunch routine by thinking outside the bag! This salad combines not only plant-based proteins, which may help improve fertility, but also fiber-rich vegetables that are loaded with antioxidants. Plus, it's simple and easy to make, meaning a stress-free meal in minutes!

Lacinato Kale Salad with Peaches and Maple Vinaigrette

MAKES: 6 servings, 1 salad each
GLUTEN FREE, VEGETARIAN, VEGAN*

Enjoy this salad as a meal by topping it with sliced Lemon Parsley Marinated Chicken (page 194), or scoop it into bowls and serve it on the side with any main dish.

1 bunch (12 ounces) lacinato kale, washed
1 teaspoon Dijon mustard
1 tablespoon maple syrup
1 tablespoon apple cider vinegar
1 teaspoon minced shallot
2 tablespoons olive oil
1 ripe peach, pitted and thinly sliced (about 1 cup)
¾ cup walnuts, toasted
½ shallot, thinly sliced
1 small (4 ounces) red bell pepper, seeded, stemmed and thinly sliced
¼ cup (1 ounce) crumbled goat cheese^{VG}
⅛ teaspoon kosher salt
⅛ teaspoon ground black pepper

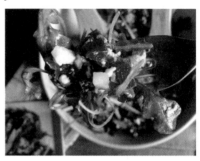

Remove the stems from the kale. Thinly slice the kale leaves and place them in a large mixing bowl. Give the kale leaves a good massage with your hands to help soften them.

To make the dressing, whisk together in a small bowl the mustard, maple syrup, apple cider vinegar, and shallot. Continue to whisk while pouring in the olive oil, mixing until combined.

Add half of the dressing to the kale and toss to coat. Let sit for about 10 minutes, then add the sliced peaches, walnuts, shallot, bell pepper, goat cheese, salt, and black pepper. Add the remaining dressing and toss. Serve immediately.

NUTRITION INFORMATION
PER SERVING: Calories 210; Fat 15g (Sat 2.5g); Protein 6g; Carb 16g; Fiber 4g; Calcium 119mg; Iron 1.6mg; Sodium 70mg; Folate 32mcg
ALLERGENS: Tree Nuts, Milk
* = Vegan Option Available

Variation: If peaches are out of season, substitute your favorite crisp apple.

Storage: Keep dressing separate if you plan to save a portion for later. Add dressing prior to assembly. Refrigerate for up to 7 days in an airtight container.

Kitchen Tip: Use chopped kale stems for a great addition to the One Pot White Bean and Kale Soup (page 165) or as a base for a homemade broth.

FERTILITY FOCUS: An easy way to increase your intake of fruits and vegetables is to pair them together. Not only do you get a sweet kick from the natural fructose present in fruits, but also a wonderful blend of nutrients, which play a crucial role in your fertility.

Panzanella with Whole Wheat Croutons

MAKES: 8 servings, 1 cup
GLUTEN FREE*, VEGETARIAN, VEGAN*

Everyone loves a delicious, crunchy crouton! We've taken that love and made it into a delicious and nutritious salad!

Croutons
¼ cup olive oil
1 clove garlic, minced
1 teaspoon Italian seasoning
¼ teaspoon kosher salt
¼ teaspoon black pepper
10 ounces whole grain bread
(or whole wheat baguette)^GF

Salad
3 tablespoons fresh lemon juice
1 clove garlic, minced
¼ cup curly parsley, chopped
¼ teaspoon kosher salt
¼ teaspoon freshly cracked black
pepper
3 tablespoons olive oil
¼ cup (1 ounce) grated Manchego
cheese (or crumbled feta cheese)^VG
1 medium (4 ounces) red onion, large
diced
1 large (6 ounces) yellow, red, or
green bell peppers, seeded,
large diced
5 medium (1 0 ounces) roma
tomatoes, cored and diced
½ cup Kalamata olives, halved
(about 21 olives)

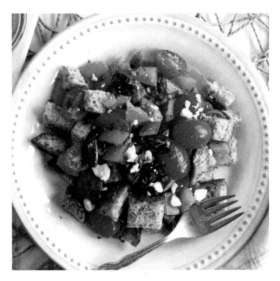

Preheat oven to 300°F and line a large baking sheet with parchment paper.

Combine the oil, garlic, Italian seasoning, salt, and pepper in a large mixing bowl. Cut the bread into 1-inch slices, then cut into 1-inch cubes and add to the bowl. Toss until evenly coated. Pour bread out onto parchment-lined baking sheet and bake 15 minutes. Stir, then bake an additional 10 minutes or until lightly golden. Set on a rack and allow to cool at least 5 minutes before serving.

In the same large mixing bowl, whisk together the lemon juice, garlic, parsley, salt, and pepper, then whisk in the olive oil.

Add the cheese, bread, onions, bell peppers, tomatoes, and olives. Toss to coat. Let stand at least 10 to 15 minutes before serving.

Variation: Substitute about 1 pint halved cherry tomatoes for the roma tomatoes.

Storage: If serving later, separate croutons from the vegetables and dressing. Add croutons 10 minutes prior to serving. Refrigerate salad mixture in an airtight container for up to 3 days. Place croutons in a sealed bag in the pantry for up to 7 days for best quality.

Kitchen Tip: If you're tight on time, grab a bag of whole wheat croutons to use in place of homemade.

NUTRITION INFORMATION
PER SERVING: Calories 260; Fat 17g (Sat 2g); Protein 7g; Carb 22g; Fiber 4g; Calcium 76mg; Iron 1.4mg; Sodium 470mg; Folate 46mcg
ALLERGENS: Wheat, Milk
* = Gluten Free, Vegan Options

FERTILITY FOCUS: Whole grains are an excellent addition to a fertility-fueling diet in many ways. Not only do they provide B vitamins, iron, and fiber, but they also help to prevent a drastic rise in your blood sugars, thus helping moderate the hormone insulin in your blood. Keeping your hormones in proper balance is crucial for achieving your most fertile self.

French Lentil Salad with Spinach and Feta

MAKES: 6 servings 1 salad each
GLUTEN FREE, VEGETARIAN, VEGAN*

A simple yet elegant salad made with green French lentils, fresh spinach, cucumbers, parsley, and feta cheese.

1 cup green or French lentils, picked over, rinsed and drained

¼ teaspoon kosher salt

2 cups (3 ounces) spinach, thinly sliced

½ cup diced red bell pepper

½ cup (1½ ounces) seeded, diced cucumber

½ cup curly parsley, finely chopped

⅓ cup crumbled feta cheese^VG

¼ cup Italian Vinaigrette (page 161, or store-bought Italian dressing)

Place lentils in a medium size pot and add enough water to cover by about 2 inches. Set pan over medium-high heat and bring to a boil. Reduce heat, cover, and simmer for about 20 minutes. Stir in salt and continue to simmer for an additional 5 to 10 minutes, or until lentils are tender. Spread on a sheet pan to cool, or rinse in cool water.

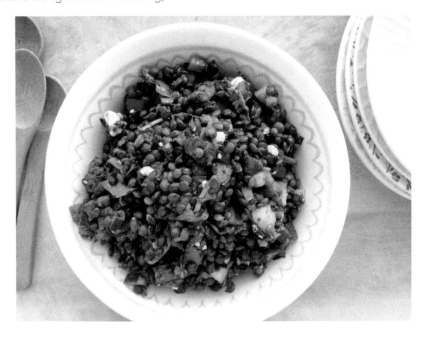

In a large salad bowl, add the cooled lentils, spinach, bell pepper, cucumber, parsley, and feta cheese. Drizzle dressing over the top and toss to combine. Serve immediately.

Storage: Keep dressing separate if you plan to save a portion for later. Add dressing prior to consumption. Refrigerate for up to 3 days in a sealed container.

NUTRITION INFORMATION
PER SERVING: Calories 170; Fat 9g (Sat 2g); Protein 8g; Carb 16g; Fiber 4g; Calcium 83mg; Iron 3mg; Sodium 190mg; Folate 59mcg
ALLERGENS: Milk
* = Vegan Option

FERTILITY FOCUS: Spinach pairs with lentils to produce a powerhouse combination, creating a perfectly satisfying meal. Serve this on its own for a light lunch, or as a side with dinner, and rest easy knowing you're well on your way to practicing what research says is a fertility-fueling diet!

SALAD DRESSINGS

Simplify your life (and your ingredient lists) by making your own salad dressings! Many of these dressings can easily be made using ingredients you already have on hand.

FERTILITY FOCUS: As you can tell, we have a strong affection for using olive oil and plain Greek yogurt in our recipes. The reason is twofold: both provide healthy fertility-boosting nutrition, and both are usually on hand in our kitchens! Preparing food at home, including dressings, means you'll be getting more wholesome, natural ingredients than if you consumed store-bought versions.

Creamy Chipotle Salad Dressing

MAKES: 6 servings, 1 tablespoon each
GLUTEN FREE, VEGETARIAN

¼ cup plain whole milk Greek yogurt
1 tablespoon chopped chipotle pepper
in adobo (or 2 teaspoons chipotle
hot sauce)

½ lime, juiced
1 tablespoon water
1 teaspoon cumin

Combine all of the ingredients in a mixing bowl and whisk to combine. Serve on salad of choice, or as a dressing on the Tex Mex Burrito Bowl (page 210).

Storage: Refrigerate in a sealed container for up to 1 week.

Shopping Tip: Pick up canned chipotle pepper in adobo in the Mexican food aisle of your local market.

NUTRITION INFORMATION
PER SERVING: Calories 15; Fat 0.5g (Sat 0g); Protein 1g; Carb 1g; Fiber 0g; Calcium 13mg; Iron 0.1mg; Sodium 15mg; Folate 0mcg
ALLERGENS: Milk

Feta Greek Yogurt Dressing

 MAKES: 6 servings, 2 tablespoons each
GLUTEN FREE, VEGETARIAN

⅔ cup plain whole milk Greek yogurt
3 tablespoons (1½ ounces) crumbled
 feta cheese
2 tablespoons white wine vinegar
1 tablespoon water

½ teaspoon garlic powder
¼ teaspoon ground black pepper
¼ teaspoon dried dill
⅛ teaspoon kosher salt

Combine all of the ingredients in a mixing bowl and whisk well to combine.

Storage: Store in a sealed container in the refrigerator for up to 1 week.

NUTRITION INFORMATION
PER SERVING: Calories 25; Fat 1.5g (Sat 1g); Protein 2g; Carb 1g; Fiber 0g; Calcium 38mg; Iron 0.1mg; Sodium
70mg; Folate 2mcg
ALLERGENS: Milk

Italian Vinaigrette

MAKES: 6 servings, 1 tablespoon each
GLUTEN FREE, VEGAN

1 teaspoon Dijon mustard
1 clove garlic, minced
2 tablespoon + 1 teaspoon red wine
 vinegar

¼ cup olive oil
1 teaspoon Italian seasoning
⅛ teaspoon kosher salt
¼ teaspoon ground black pepper

In the bottom of a small mixing bowl, combine the mustard, garlic, and vinegar. Whisk in
the olive oil and stir until combined. Add the Italian seasoning, salt, and pepper, and mix.

Storage: Store in a sealed container in the refrigerator for up to 1 week.

NUTRITION INFORMATION
PER SERVING: Calories 80; Fat 9g (Sat 1g); Protein 0g; Carb 0g; Fiber 0g; Calcium 2mg; Iron 0.1mg; Sodium 60mg;
Folate 0mcg

Maple Vinaigrette

MAKES: 12 servings, 1 tablespoon each
GLUTEN FREE, VEGAN

1 tablespoon Dijon mustard
3 tablespoons maple syrup
3 tablespoons apple cider vinegar
1 tablespoon minced shallot
¼ cup + 2 tablespoons olive oil

In a small bowl, whisk together the mustard, maple syrup, apple cider vinegar, and shallot. Whisk in the olive oil, mixing until combined.

Storage: Store in a sealed container in the refrigerator for up to 1 week.

NUTRITION INFORMATION
PER SERVING: Calories 70; Fat 7g (Sat 1g); Protein 0g; Carb 4g; Fiber 0g; Calcium 6mg; Iron 0.1mg; Sodium 30mg; Folate 0.3mcg

Champagne Vinaigrette

MAKES: 8 servings, 1 tablespoon each
GLUTEN FREE, VEGETARIAN

1 tablespoon + 1 teaspoon Dijon
    mustard
2 teaspoons honey
2 tablespoons champagne vinegar
¼ cup olive oil
¼ teaspoon dried thyme leaves
¼ teaspoon ground black pepper

In a small bowl, whisk together the mustard, honey, and vinegar. Whisk in the olive oil, then add dried thyme and black pepper.

Storage: Store in a sealed container in the refrigerator for up to 1 week.

NUTRITION INFORMATION
PER SERVING: Calories 70; Fat 7g (Sat 1g); Protein 0g; Carb 2g; Fiber 0g; Calcium 1mg; Iron 0.1mg; Sodium 75mg; Folate 0.1mcg

Honey Lime Vinaigrette

MAKES: 10 servings, 1 tablespoon each
GLUTEN FREE, VEGETARIAN

1 teaspoon Dijon mustard
1 lime, zested and juiced (about 1
    teaspoon zest + 3 tablespoons juice)
2 tablespoons honey
⅓ cup olive oil
⅛ teaspoon kosher salt

In a small bowl, whisk together the mustard, lime zest, lime juice, and honey. Whisk in the olive oil, then add salt.

Storage: Store in a sealed container in the refrigerator for up to 1 week.

NUTRITION INFORMATION
PER SERVING: Calories 80; Fat 7g (Sat 1g); Protein 0g; Carb 4g; Fiber 0g; Calcium 1mg; Iron 0.1mg; Sodium 35mg; Folate 1mcg

Tahini Vinaigrette

MAKES: 8 servings, 1 tablespoon
GLUTEN FREE, VEGETARIAN

1 clove garlic, minced
1 tablespoon tahini
2 tablespoons fresh lemon juice
1 teaspoon honey
1 tablespoon olive oil
1 tablespoon water
⅛ teaspoon kosher salt
¼ teaspoon ground black pepper

In a mixing bowl, whisk together the garlic, tahini, lemon juice, and honey. Add the olive oil and continue whisking until combined, then add the water. Season with salt and pepper.

Storage: Store in a sealed container in the refrigerator for up to 1 week.

Shopping Tip: Tahini is a ground sesame seed paste found in the international food aisle at the grocery store. It is usually in a jar and needs to be refrigerated after opening.

NUTRITION INFORMATION
PER SERVING: Calories 60; Fat 5g (Sat 0.5g); Protein 1g; Carb 3g; Fiber 0g; Calcium 8mg; Iron 0.2mg; Sodium 65mg; Folate 5mcg

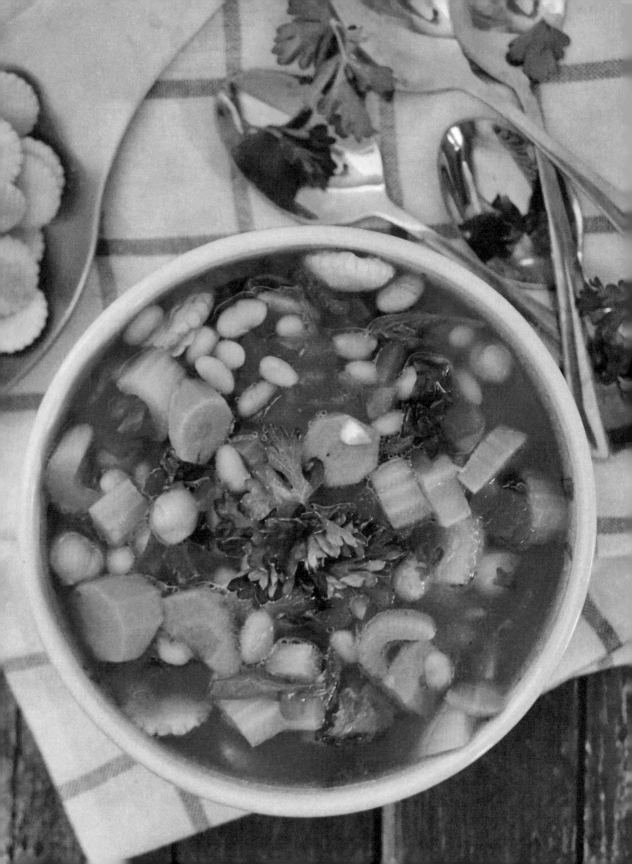

One Pot White Bean and Kale Soup

MAKES: 6 servings, 1½ to 1¾ cups each
GLUTEN FREE, VEGAN

Oh kale yeah! You didn't think you'd get through this book without us throwing some kale at you, did you? This hearty soup is a great source of nutrition and packs a ton of heart-healthy fiber.

1 tablespoon olive oil
⅓ cup (2 ounces) chopped onion
2 cups (8 ounces) chopped carrots (about 2 medium carrots)
1 cup (3 ounces) chopped celery stalks (about 2 celery stalks)
3 cloves garlic, minced
4 cups low sodium vegetable broth
1 bay leaf
2 tablespoons chopped fresh thyme
2 cans (15 ounces each) no salt added white beans, rinsed and drained
1 can (14½ ounces) no salt added diced tomatoes
2 cups (2½ ounces) baby kale
½ teaspoon ground black pepper
¼ teaspoon kosher salt
¼ cup fresh parsley, chopped

Set a large pot over medium heat and add olive oil. Once hot, add onion, carrots, and celery and stir until tender, about 8 to 10 minutes. Add the garlic and cook an additional minute. Add the vegetable broth, bay leaf, and white beans to the pot. Cover with lid and simmer over low heat for 20 minutes.

Turn heat to low and add the baby kale, black pepper, and salt. Cover and continue cooking about 10 minutes, or until kale is tender.

Remove bay leaf, portion into bowls, garnish with parsley and enjoy.

Shopping Tip: Pick up baby kale in the prepackaged produce section. Or use an equal amount of chopped kale.

Storage: Refrigerate in a sealed container for up 4 days. Freeze for up to 3 months.

NUTRITION INFORMATION
PER SERVING: Calories 200; Fat 3g (Sat 0g); Protein 10g; Carb 37g; Fiber 11g; Calcium 178mg; Iron 3.2mg; Sodium 510mg; Folate 161mcg

FERTILITY FOCUS: Plant-based proteins, like legumes, are an excellent way to fuel your fertility while providing dietary fiber and essential vitamins and minerals. Research suggests that higher rates of conception occur with those who follow a predominantly plant-based diet.

Chicken Pozole

  MAKES: 6 servings of 1⅓ cups each
GLUTEN FREE*

Pozole is a comforting bowl of warmth and goodness, and ours is meant to be just that! Serve yourself up a bowl of this satisfying soup for lunch or dinner.

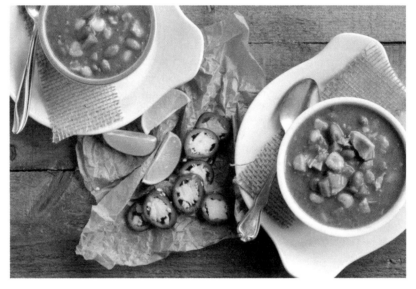

1 tablespoon vegetable oil
2 skin-on, bone-in chicken thighs
   (about ¾ pound)
2 skin-on, bone-in chicken breasts
   (about 1¼ pound)
1 cup (4½ ounces) diced onion
1 cup (5 ounces) diced carrots
1 tablespoon chili powder
1 teaspoon ground cumin
¼ cup white whole wheat flour^{GF}

4 cups low sodium chicken broth
1 can (15½ ounces) no salt added pinto
   beans, rinsed and drained
1 can (25 ounces) hominy, drained
   (about 1¾ cup drained)
1 can (4 ounces) diced green chiles
1 lime, juiced (about 2 tablespoons)
½ cup fresh cilantro, chopped
Salt, to taste

Heat oil in a large pot or Dutch oven over medium-high heat until shimmering. Arrange chicken, skin side down, in the pot. Sear chicken 7 to 8 minutes, or until skin is golden brown. Move to a plate and reserve. Remove 1 tablespoon of fat and discard.

Add the onion and carrots to the pot and cook, stirring often, until softened, about 6 to 7 minutes. Add the chili powder and cumin and cook, stirring until fragrant, about 1 minute. Stir in the flour and cook for another minute. Add the chicken broth, stirring to scrape any bits off the bottom of the pan. Bring mixture to a simmer, then add the chicken, pressing it into the liquid to fully submerge it.

Reduce heat to medium-low and simmer, partially covered, until chicken is cooked (165°F), about 25 to 30 minutes. Check occasionally during cooking to ensure that chicken is still submerged. Add water, ½ cup at a time, to keep chicken in the cooking liquid.

Move the chicken to a cutting board and let it cool for 5 minutes. At this point, you can also skim the surface of the soup to remove any excess fat.

Carefully remove and discard skin. Using a fork, remove the meat from the bones. Discard bones. Roughly chop the chicken and add it back to the pot, along with the drained beans, hominy, and chiles. Cook an additional 10 minutes. Stir in lime juice and cilantro. Season to taste.

Variation: To spice things up, add some sliced jalapeño before serving.

Storage: Refrigerate in a sealed container for up to 4 days. Freeze for up to 3 months.

NUTRITION INFORMATION

PER SERVING: Calories 350; Fat 13g (Sat 3g); Protein 30g; Carb 29g; Fiber 6g; Calcium 100mg; Iron 3.1mg; Sodium 790mg; Folate 49mcg

ALLERGEN: Wheat

* = Gluten Free Option

FERTILITY FOCUS: Stress is often related to infertility. That means finding ways to unwind and let go of the stress of the day is essential to achieving a balanced state of well-being. We enjoy taking time to cook hearty, nutrient-dense meals like this as part of our stress relief therapy. Turn on the music and let yourself enjoy "cooking therapy!"

Red Lentil Curry Soup

  MAKES: 6 servings of 1¼ cups each
GLUTEN FREE, VEGAN

Loaded with warm spices, this soup is both rich and satisfying. Red lentils cook quickly and add a touch of earthiness, which is complemented by the brightness of the lemon juice.

1 tablespoon olive oil
1 small (2½ ounces) onion, chopped
   (about ⅔ cup)
4 cloves garlic, minced
2 tablespoons minced fresh ginger (or 1
   teaspoon ground ginger)
1½ tablespoons curry powder
1½ teaspoons ground cumin
1 teaspoon ground cinnamon

1½ cup red lentils (picked over to
   remove debris or rocks and rinsed)
4 cups low sodium vegetable broth
2 cups water
¼ cup lemon juice
¼ teaspoon kosher salt
¼ cup chopped fresh cilantro
Sriracha, to taste

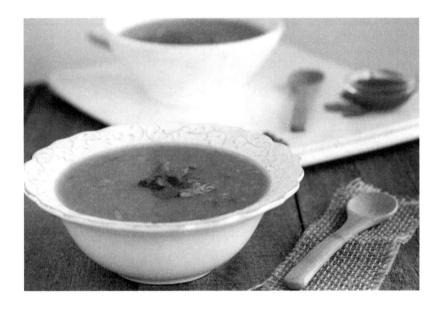

Place a large pot over medium heat and add the olive oil. Add onions and sauté until softened, about 5 minutes. Add garlic, ginger, curry, cumin, and cinnamon, and sauté 1 minute. Add the lentils and cook 1 minute more. Stir in the vegetable broth and water and bring to a simmer. Turn the heat to medium low and allow the soup to simmer, partially covered, for about 30 minutes or until the lentils are cooked.

Take the soup off of the heat. Remove half of the soup and allow it to cool slightly, keeping the other half warm on the stove. Place the cooled soup in a blender or use an immersion blender and pulse until pureed. Stir pureed mixture back into the pot of soup and turn the flame back to medium. Add the lemon juice and salt and stir.

To serve, place the soup in bowls and garnish with cilantro and Sriracha.

Variations:

- If the soup is too spicy, decrease the amount of curry powder and add a little more turmeric, or purchase a less spicy curry powder.
- Lemon juice adds flavor and depth without added salt. It can easily be replaced with red wine vinegar. Start with 1 tablespoon and taste before adding more.
- While fresh ginger is best for this recipe, it can be replaced with ground ginger. Substitute about ¼ teaspoon ground ginger for the 2 tablespoons fresh in this recipe.

Storage: Refrigerate in a sealed container for up to 4 days. Freeze for up to 3 months.

Shopping Tip: Red lentils can be found in the health food aisle at your local supermarket (sometimes they'll be in the international aisle, as well).

Kitchen Tip: It is not advised to puree hot items in a blender due to the build-up of pressure generated by the steam. Be safe and allow your soup to cool slightly to prevent injuring yourself.

NUTRITION INFORMATION
One serving: Calories 220; Fat 3.5g (Sat .5g); Protein 12g; Carb 36g; Fiber 7g; Calcium 62mg; Iron 4.4mg; Sodium 190mg; Folate 103mcg

---

FERTILITY FOCUS: Replacing meat proteins with legumes may promote fertility. Focusing on incorporating more meatless meals throughout your week is a great way to add variety while also providing fiber, folate, and magnesium!

Thai Peanut Carrot Soup

MAKES: 4 servings, 1 cup each
GLUTEN FREE, VEGAN

This soup is anything but short on flavor—fresh ginger, garlic, and peanut butter build upon well-loved Thai cuisine flavors. Trust us, it is addicting, so be mindful of your portion size . . . even though you may want to eat the whole bowl!

1 tablespoon olive oil
1 pound carrots, peeled and chopped (about 3 cups chopped)
1¼ cup (5½ ounces) diced yellow onion
2 rounded tablespoons (24 grams) peeled, chopped fresh ginger
2 cloves garlic, chopped
3 cups low sodium vegetable broth
¼ cup Natural Peanut Butter (page 59), or store bought creamy peanut butter
3 tablespoons fresh lime juice
¼ teaspoon kosher salt
¼ cup cilantro, roughly chopped
¼ cup peanuts, chopped
3 to 5 Thai bird chiles, thinly sliced (or jalapenos or serrano peppers)

Set a large pot over medium-high heat and add the oil. Once hot, add the carrots and onion and cook until softened, stirring often, about 8 to 10 minutes. Add ginger and garlic and cook for 1 minute, stirring constantly. Add broth and bring to a boil. Reduce the heat to a simmer, partially cover, and cook until vegetables are tender, about 30 minutes.

Remove pot from the heat and cool slightly. Puree in batches, then return to the pot. Stir in the peanut butter and lime juice. Season with salt.

Portion into bowls and garnish with cilantro, peanuts, and Thai chiles.

Storage: Refrigerate in a sealed container for up to 4 days. Freeze for up to 3 months.

Shopping Tip: Find Thai chiles in the produce section of your market, near the spicy peppers.

NUTRITION INFORMATION
PER SERVING: Calories 290; Fat 17g (Sat 2.5g); Protein 9g; Carb 27g; Fiber 7g; Calcium 77mg; Iron 0.9mg; Sodium 360mg; Folate 39mcg
ALLERGENS: Peanuts

FERTILITY FOCUS: Filled with carrots, this soup provides a powerful punch of anti-oxidants. Antioxidants are compounds in food that keep your body functioning at its best. Research shows that higher intakes of antioxidant foods helps increase your chances of fertility (see Chapter 3), so grab a spoon and dive in with us!

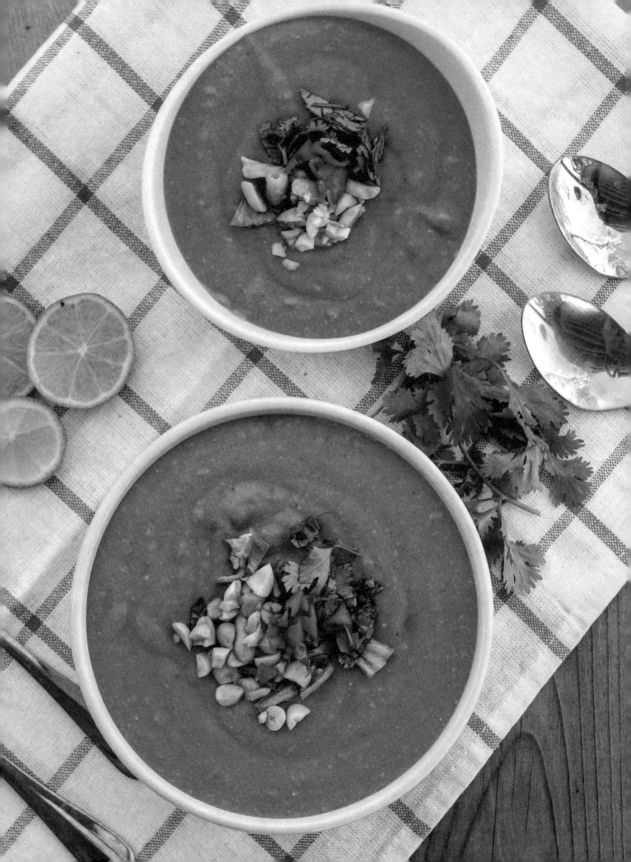

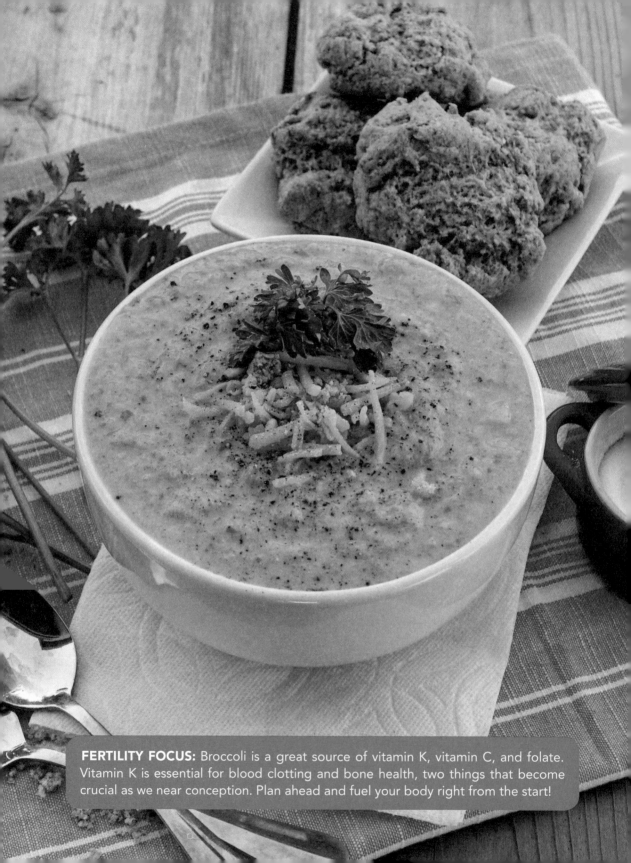

FERTILITY FOCUS: Broccoli is a great source of vitamin K, vitamin C, and folate. Vitamin K is essential for blood clotting and bone health, two things that become crucial as we near conception. Plan ahead and fuel your body right from the start!

Broccoli Cheese Soup

 MAKES: 5 servings of 1 cup each
GLUTEN FREE*, VEGETARIAN

Cheesy soups can fit in a fertility-filled diet! This twist on Broccoli Cheese Soup is loaded with flavor, filling fiber, and lots of love, just what you need right now. Grab a bowl with a Whole Wheat Biscuit (page 234) and unwind after a long day.

1 large head broccoli (about 1¼ pounds)
3 tablespoons olive oil
¾ cup (3¼ ounces) diced white or yellow onion
¼ cup (1 ounce) diced carrot
¼ cup (1 ounce) diced celery
1 clove garlic, minced
3 tablespoons white whole wheat flour^{GF}
1 cup whole milk
2½ cups low sodium vegetable broth
1 cup shredded sharp cheddar cheese
2 teaspoons white wine vinegar
½ teaspoon kosher salt
¼ teaspoon black pepper

Wash broccoli and remove the stems and stalk from the head. Peel the stem and stalk to remove the tough, outer parts, then finely chop. Chop florets separately and reserve.

Heat the oil in a large pot over medium heat. Add the broccoli stems, stalk, onion, carrot, and celery. Cook until softened, stirring frequently, about 8 to 10 minutes. Add the garlic and cook 1 minute more.

Stir in the flour and cook 3 to 4 minutes, until golden. Whisk in the milk. Add the broth and bring to a simmer, partially cover and cook until slightly thickened, about 10 minutes.

Remove from heat and cool slightly. Puree in batches, then return to the pot. Add broccoli florets and cook an additional 5 to 10 minutes, or until tender (puree the mixture again at this point if a smoother soup is desired).

Stir in the cheese and white wine vinegar and mix until melted. Season with salt and pepper and serve immediately.

Storage: Refrigerate in a sealed container for up to 4 days. Freeze for up to 3 months.

NUTRITION INFORMATION
PER SERVING: Calories 260; Fat 17g (Sat 6g); Protein 11g; Carb 18mg; Fiber 5g; Calcium 281mg; Iron 1.3mg; Sodium 480mg; Folate 132mcg
ALLERGENS: Wheat, Milk
* = Gluten Free Option

Classic Chicken Noodle Soup

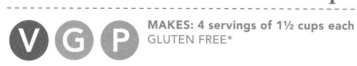

MAKES: 4 servings of 1½ cups each
GLUTEN FREE*

Nothing says comfort like a bowl of homemade chicken soup. After the tenth doctor's visit of the month, sometimes you just need a familiar classic. This soup is just that, and it's made in a crock pot so you can walk in the door and know dinner is served!

½ medium (4 ounces) onion, chopped
1 cup (6 ounces) carrots, chopped
1 cup (6 ounces) celery, chopped
3 cloves garlic, minced
1 pound boneless, skinless chicken breasts
2 teaspoons dried oregano leaves

1 teaspoon ground black pepper
⅛ teaspoon kosher salt
2 bay leaves
4 cups low sodium vegetable broth
1 cup dry whole wheat bow tie pasta (or alternative whole wheat short pasta)GF

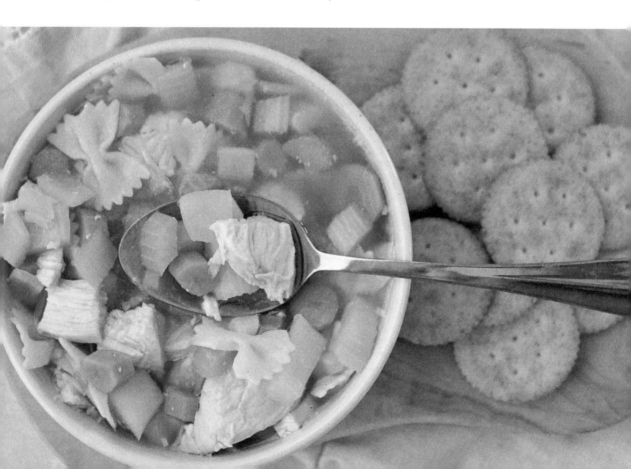

Add the onions, carrots, celery, and garlic to a 3- to 4-quart slow cooker. Place the chicken on top with the oregano, black pepper, salt, bay leaves, and vegetable broth. Set to low, cover, and cook for 4 hours.

Remove lid and add pasta. Cook an additional 30 minutes on low. Remove and discard bay leaves. Using two forks, shred the chicken breast. Caution: it will be hot!

Serve immediately with a Whole Wheat Biscuit (page 234) or side salad.

Storage: Refrigerate in a sealed container for up to 4 days. Freeze for up to 3 months.

NUTRITION INFORMATION
PER SERVING: Calories 280; Fat 3.5g (Sat 1g); Protein 30g; Carb 31g; Fiber 6g; Calcium 86mg; Iron 2.2mg; Sodium 310mg; Folate 38mcg
ALLERGENS: Wheat
* = Gluten Free Option

FERTILITY FOCUS: Filled with vegetables and nourishing lean protein, this soup is just what your doctor ordered. Plus, by making this yourself, you control the salt content. Too much salt can raise your blood pressure and increase your risk of cardiovascular disease.

Tomato Vegetable Soup

MAKES: 5 servings of 1 cup each
GLUTEN FREE, VEGETARIAN, VEGAN*

Tomato soup gets a facelift with this new twist on a classic! Make a batch and serve alongside the Broiled Tomato and Sharp Cheddar Grilled Cheese (page 118) for an excellent meal in minutes!

1 cup (4½ ounces) yellow onion, chopped
½ cup (2½ ounces) carrots, peeled and chopped
½ cup (2 ounces) chopped celery
2 cloves garlic, chopped
2 tablespoons tomato paste
1 can (28 ounces) diced tomatoes, no salt added
2 cups low sodium vegetable broth

1 dried bay leaf
1 tablespoon + 1 teaspoon red wine vinegar
¼ teaspoon crushed red pepper flakes (or ⅛ teaspoon for less heat)
¼ cup fresh basil, chopped
1 tablespoon packed brown sugar
½ teaspoon kosher salt
⅓ cup shredded Parmesan cheese^{VG}

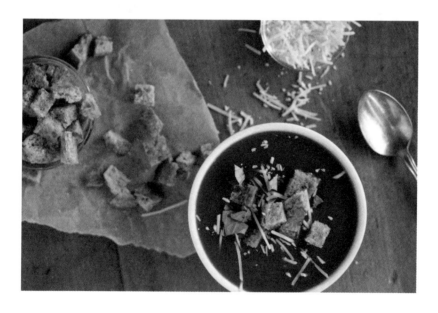

Place the onion, carrots, celery, garlic, tomato paste, diced tomatoes, vegetable broth, and bay leaf in a 3- to 4-quart slow cooker that's been sprayed with cooking spray. Stir to combine. Cover with the lid and cook on low for 6 to 7 hours, or on high for 4 hours.

Remove and discard the bay leaf. Add the vinegar, crushed red pepper, basil, brown sugar, and salt, and puree with an immersion blender until smooth. Cover with lid and cook an additional 30 minutes.

Portion into bowls and garnish with Parmesan cheese.

Variation: Stir in your favorite mix-ins to make this a "loaded" bowl of soup. For a pizza soup, stir in turkey pepperoni, or try ham, bell peppers, and olives. For a taco soup, stir in cooked chicken, black beans, corn, Mexican cheese, and top with avocado.

Storage: Refrigerate in a sealed container for up to 4 days. Freeze for up to 3 months.

Kitchen Tip: In place of an immersion blender, puree in batches using your blender, covering the hole with a towel to allow steam to escape.

NUTRITION INFORMATION
PER SERVING: Calories 100; Fat 1.5g (Sat 1g); Protein 4g; Carb 17g; Fiber 4g; Calcium 124mg; Iron 1.1mg; Sodium 470mg; Folate 11mcg
ALLERGENS: Milk
* = Vegan Option

FERTILITY FOCUS: The star of this recipe, the beautiful tomato, is an excellent addition to a fertility diet. It's filled with lycopene, that stellar antioxidant that shows promise of increasing fertility in men and helps naturally rid the body of free radicals.

Smoky Sweet Potato Chili

  MAKES: 7 servings of 1 cup each
GLUTEN FREE, VEGAN

Warm up with this smoky and slightly spicy vegan, gluten free chili. It tastes great on its own, but is also wonderful when topped with the No Fail Guacamole (page 116) and served with a side of Oven Baked Tortilla Chips (page 112).

½ medium onion (4 ounces), finely chopped
2 cloves garlic, minced
1 small jalapeño, seeded and minced
2 medium (3 ounces, 1 cup) carrots, diced
1 (½ cup) green bell pepper, seeded and diced
1 medium (9 ounces) sweet potato, washed, peeled, diced into ¼-inch cubes
1 (28 ounce) can diced tomatoes, no added salt
½ cup water

1 teaspoon chili powder
2 teaspoon smoked paprika
1 teaspoon ground cumin
¼ teaspoon kosher salt
1 can (15½ ounces) no salt added black beans, drained and rinsed
1 can (15½ ounces) no salt added pinto beans, drained and rinsed
1 medium avocado, sliced (garnish)
¼ cup chopped cilantro (optional garnish)

Place the onion, garlic, jalapeño, carrot, bell pepper, and sweet potato on the bottom of the slow cooker. Stir in the diced tomatoes, water, chili powder, paprika, cumin, and salt.

Set slow cooker to low, cover, and cook for 3 to 4 hours. Add the pinto and black beans 10 minutes prior to serving.

Before serving, garnish with sliced avocado and chopped cilantro.

Variation: Add 1 tablespoon of Creamy Chipotle Salad Dressing (page 160) to finish dish.

Storage: Refrigerate in a sealed container for up to 4 days. Freeze for up to 3 months.

Kitchen Tip: Wash sweet potatoes by using a paper towel under running water. Rub until debris and dirt is removed.

NUTRITION INFORMATION
PER SERVING: Calories 210; Fat 3g (Sat 0g); Protein 9g; Carb 40g; Fiber 12g; Calcium 102mg; Iron 3.2mg; Sodium 340mg; Folate 77mcg

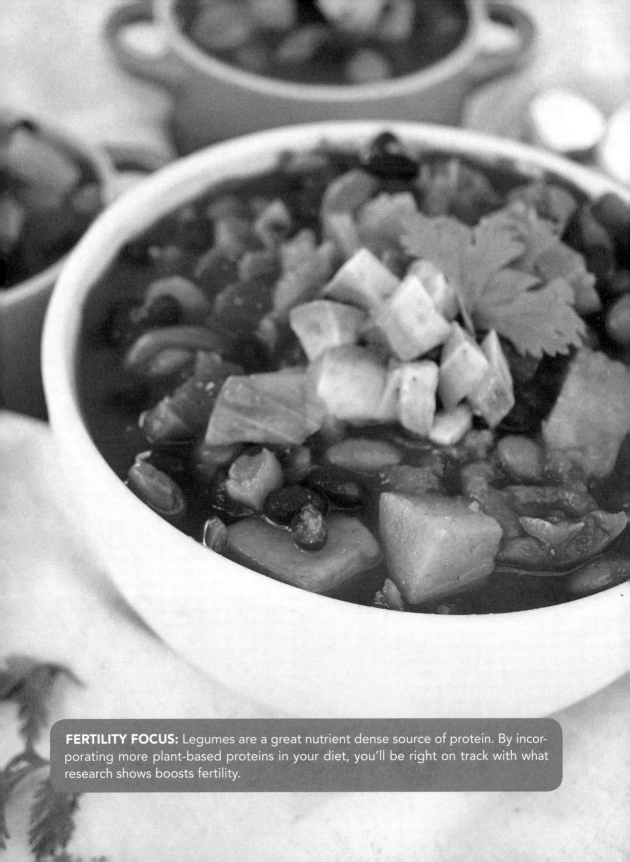

FERTILITY FOCUS: Legumes are a great nutrient dense source of protein. By incorporating more plant-based proteins in your diet, you'll be right on track with what research shows boosts fertility.

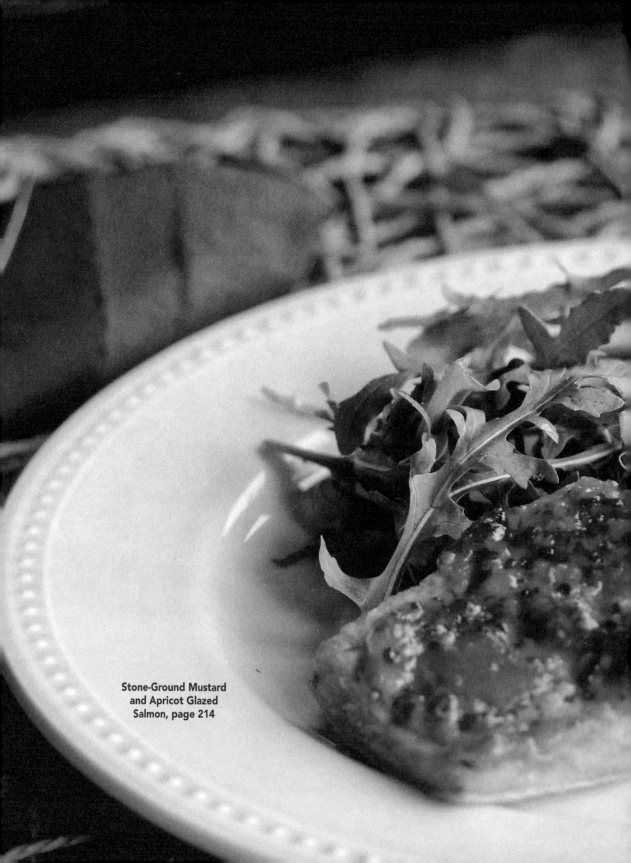

Stone-Ground Mustard
and Apricot Glazed
Salmon, page 214

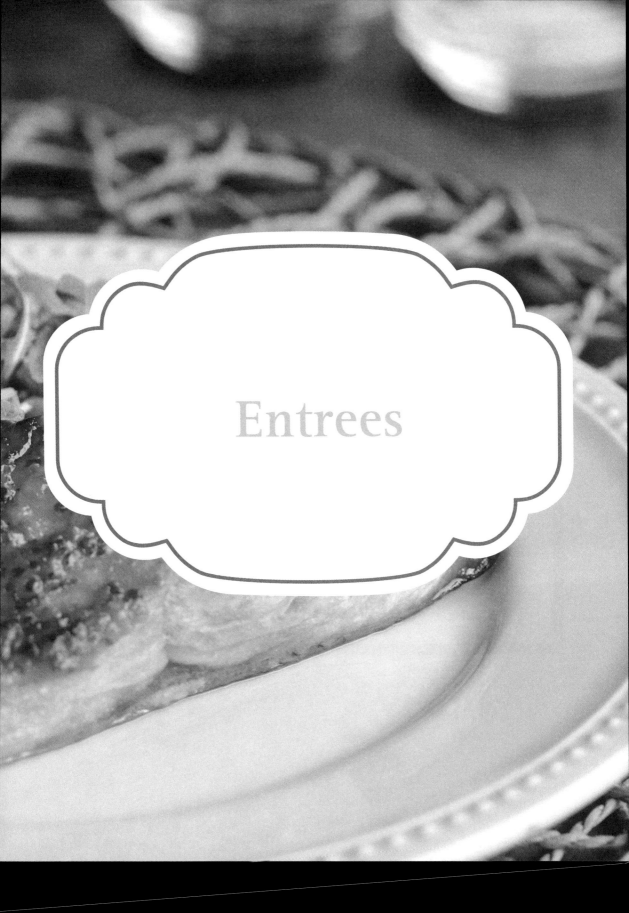

Entrees

THINKING ABOUT WHAT TO eat for dinner can be overwhelming, right? We agree—that's why we've done the work for you! This section gives you creative menu ideas to implement as part of your weekly routine. Plus, we've given you a variety of recipes and cuisines, so regardless of what you have in your house or what you're craving that week, there's bound to be a recipe for you!

Looking for more ideas? We've compiled a list of some simple meals to provide nourishment without fuss.

STAPLE FOOD	SIMPLE FERTILITY FUEL MEAL
Quinoa	Reheat some frozen quinoa and add it to a salad or cooked, frozen veggies. Or, use it as the base for your next "bowl" meal and top with your favorite vegetables and beans.
Eggs	Breakfast for dinner is a great quick fix meal. Scramble two eggs and serve with a slice of whole grain toast topped with avocado and a side of fruit.
Beans	Open a can of your favorite beans, then rinse and drain, and you've got yourself a fiber filled plant based protein. Or, take out those Mexican Black Beans from Scratch (page 242). Wrap beans in corn tortillas with shredded cabbage, salsa and cheese and voila, dinner is served!
Quesadillas	Use a whole grain tortilla to create a simple quesadilla. This versatile meal provides a serving of whole grains and dairy, as well as protein and vegetables. Here's some recipe inspiration to jazz up your quesadilla: • Spread Garlic Hummus (page 103) and top with roasted peppers and feta cheese. • Add black beans and cheddar cheese and top with Guacamole (page 116) and Pico de Gallo Salsa (page 114). • Fill with spinach and mozzarella cheese then top with Homemade Marinara Sauce (page 184).

Parmesan Pesto Pasta with Cherry Tomatoes

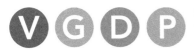

MAKES: 8 servings, 1½ cups each
GLUTEN FREE*, VEGETARIAN

In need of a recipe for a hot summer day? Are you looking for a great dish to bring to a potluck? This Pesto Pasta Salad is the perfect dish for nearly every occasion.

1 pound whole wheat bowtie pasta (or bite size pasta of choice)GF
½ cup Pesto Sauce (page 186) or store bought pesto
1 cup cherry tomatoes, halved
4 cups (2 ounces) baby spinach leaves
1 cup (7 ounces) chopped roasted red peppers
¼ cup grated Parmesan cheese
¼ teaspoon kosher salt
½ teaspoon crushed red pepper
Basil, thinly sliced, for garnish

Cook pasta according to package directions. Drain, place in a large bowl, and immediately toss with the prepared pesto. Add the cherry tomatoes, spinach, roasted red peppers, Parmesan cheese, salt, and crushed red pepper. Toss to combine. Serve immediately.

Variation: Add lean protein by including some Slow Cooker Pulled Chicken (page 196).

Storage: Refrigerate in a sealed container for up to 4 days. For best quality, do not freeze.

Shopping Tip: Pre-made pesto can be found in the refrigerated deli section or by the pasta sauces. Roasted red bell peppers can be found on the condiment aisle or Italian section at your local market.

Kitchen Tip: Portion the pasta in individual containers and use as a quick grab-and-go lunch option.

NUTRITION INFORMATION
PER SERVING: Calories 330; Fat 12g (Sat 2.5g); Protein 14g; Carb 45g; Fiber 6g; Calcium 189mg; Iron 3.3mg; Sodium 280mg; Folate 82mcg
ALLERGENS: Wheat, Tree Nuts, Milk
* = Gluten Free Option

FERTILITY FOCUS: Whole grains, healthy fats, and fiber filling vegetables combine to provide the ultimate fertility fueling meal. Whole grains help stabilize those blood sugars, while lycopene is a stellar antioxidant; both are crucial in achieving your most fertile self.

Homemade Marinara Sauce

MAKES: 5 cups, 10 servings, ½ cup each
GLUTEN FREE, VEGAN

A simple marinara sauce that's perfect for pizza or tossed with pasta.

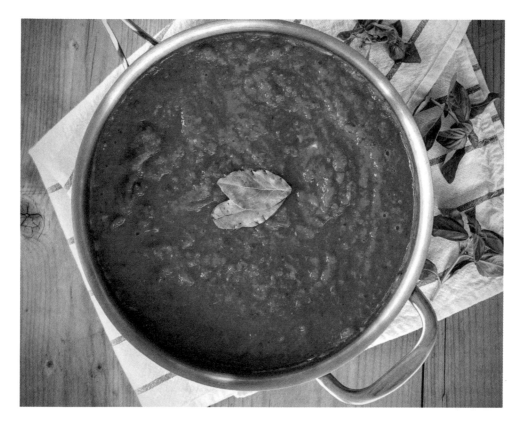

1 tablespoon olive oil
1 medium (10 ounces) onion, diced
1 medium (7 ounces) red or yellow bell
   pepper, diced
1 medium (7 ounces) green bell
   pepper, diced
2 cloves garlic, minced
1 tablespoon tomato paste

1 can (28 ounces) diced tomatoes,
   solids and liquids
¼ cup water
2 tablespoons red wine vinegar
1 teaspoon Italian seasoning
1 bay leaf
1 tablespoon brown sugar
¼ teaspoon kosher salt

Heat the oil in a deep-sided sauté pan set over medium-high heat. Once the oil is hot, add the onion and peppers. Cook, stirring frequently, until vegetables are slightly tender, about 10 to 12 minutes. Add the garlic and cook 1 more minute. Stir in the tomato paste and cook for 3 more minutes.

Add the can of diced tomatoes, water, and vinegar. Stir, scraping the bottom of the pan to lift any ingredient residue that sticks. Add the Italian seasoning, bay leaf, and brown sugar. Bring to a boil, then reduce the heat to a simmer. Cover and cook for 30 minutes to 1 hour.

Remove and discard the bay leaf and add the salt. Using an immersion blender, carefully puree the mixture until smooth. Alternatively, work in batches using a blender or food processor, exercising caution with the hot mixture (follow manufacturer's instructions for pureeing hot or warm ingredients).

Storage: Refrigerate in a sealed container for 3 days or freeze for up to 2 months.

NUTRITION INFORMATION
PER SERVING: Calories 60; Fat 0g (Sat 0g); Protein 1g; Carb 10g; Fiber 2g; Calcium 23mg; Iron 1mg; Sodium 240mg; Folate 13mcg

FERTILITY FOCUS: This sauce is filled with lycopene, a stellar phytonutrient that has been shown to help rid your body of those free radicals that can inhibit both male and female infertility.

Spinach Pesto Sauce

 MAKES: ¾ cup, 36 servings, 1 teaspoon each
GLUTEN FREE, VEGETARIAN

Pesto sauce is remade with a healthy, green twist! We recommend pairing this Spinach Pesto Sauce with the Parmesan Pesto Pasta with Cherry Tomatoes (page 183) or using it as a unique spread on one of our sandwiches (pages 117–129).

2 cups (1¼ ounces) lightly packed basil leaves
1 cup (1 ounce) packed baby spinach leaves
3 cloves garlic, smashed
¼ cup (1 ounce) toasted pine nuts

⅓ cup + 1 tablespoon olive oil
2 tablespoon water
½ cup grated Parmesan cheese
¼ teaspoon ground black pepper
¼ teaspoon kosher salt

In the bowl of a blender or food processor, add basil, spinach, garlic, and pine nuts, and pulse until finely chopped, scraping down the sides as needed. Slowly stream in the olive oil, then add water and blend until smooth. Add the cheese, pepper, and salt and pulse 2 to 3 times.

Use pesto immediately or put in a clean container and cover with a thin layer (approximately 1 tablespoon) of olive oil to prevent it from browning.

Variation: Substitute ⅓ cup chopped walnut for pine nuts.

Storage: Refrigerate in a sealed container for 3 days or freeze (omitting cheese) for up to 2 months.

Kitchen Tip: Place in ice cubes trays to freeze. Enjoy as an easy and flavorful addition to soups.

NUTRITION INFORMATION
PER SERVING: Calories 35; Fat 3.5g (Sat 0.5g); Protein 1g; Carb 0g; Fiber 0g; Calcium 29mg; Iron 0.2mg; Sodium 45mg; Folate 5mcg
ALLERGENS: Tree Nuts, Milk

FERTILITY FOCUS: Healthy fats from the pine nuts (or walnuts) combine with fresh basil and olive oil to leave you feeling satiated from this homemade pesto. Enjoy every bite knowing you are providing your body with a bit more nutrition (fiber, phytonutrients and vitamin K) from the stealth health move of adding spinach. We told you, we love our veggies!

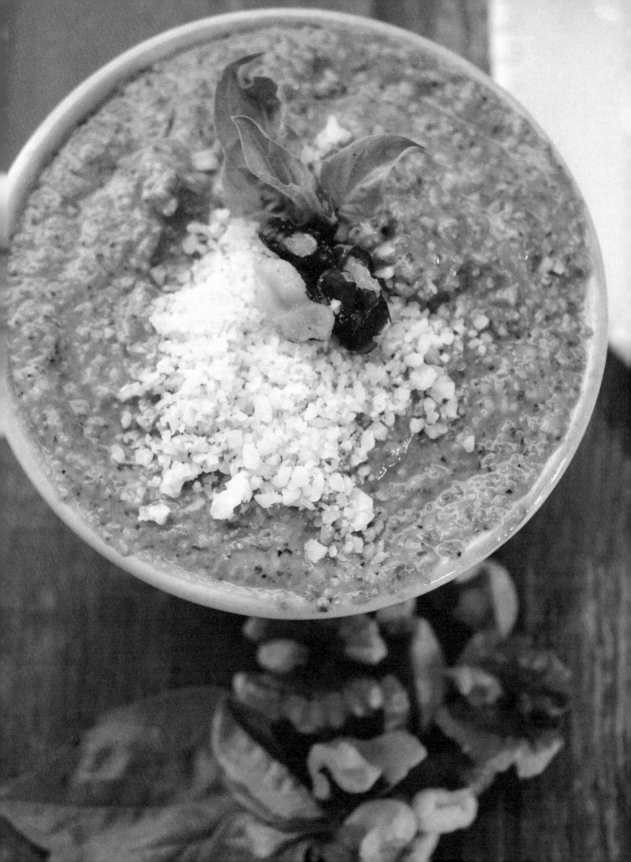

3-Cheese Baked Penne Lasagna with Fresh Arugula Salad

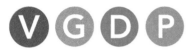 **MAKES: 8 servings, 1 serving each**
GLUTEN FREE*, VEGETARIAN

A fun twist on a favorite! This one includes fresh arugula sprinkled over the top, adding a refreshing, crisp bite.

Pasta
1 pound whole wheat penne pasta[GF]
3 cups Marinara Sauce (page 184) or
    3 cups store bought pasta sauce
1 cup whole milk ricotta cheese
4 tablespoons grated Parmesan cheese,
    divided
½ cup whole milk shredded mozzarella
    cheese

Arugula Salad
4 cups (4 ounces) fresh arugula, loosely
    packed
2 teaspoons olive oil
¼ teaspoon ground black pepper

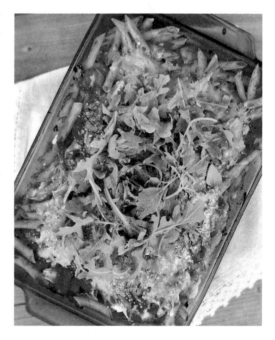

Preheat oven to 400°F and coat a 9 x 13-inch baking pan with cooking spray.

Cook pasta according to package instructions, cooking to al dente or still slightly toothsome.

Drain, then add the marinara sauce, stirring to combine. Pour half of the pasta with sauce into the prepared pan and spread the ricotta cheese over the top. Sprinkle 2 tablespoons of Parmesan cheese over the ricotta. Cover with the remaining pasta. Sprinkle with mozzarella cheese and remaining Parmesan cheese.

Bake for 20 to 25 minutes. Remove from oven and let rest at least 10 minutes. Just before serving, combine the arugula, olive oil and black pepper. Sprinkle over the top of each serving.

Variation: Swap kale or spinach for the arugula.

Storage: Refrigerate in a sealed container for 4 days or freeze for up to 2 months.

NUTRITION INFORMATION
PER SERVING: Calories 330; Fat 10g (Sat 4.5g); Protein 16g; Carb 49g; Fiber 6g; Calcium 211mg; Iron 2.5mg; Sodium 300mg; Folate 34mcg
ALLERGENS: Wheat, Milk
* = Gluten Free Option

FERTILITY FOCUS: Whole grain pasta is an excellent way to increase your intake of B vitamins and fiber. Research supports increasing whole grains in your daily diet to help with fertility and stabilizing your blood sugars.

Greek Pasta Salad

 MAKES: 8 servings, 1½ cups each
GLUTEN FREE*, VEGETARIAN

A simple yet delicious cold pasta salad that is perfect on its own or tastes wonderful as a side to the Marinated Chicken (page 194).

Pasta Salad

12 ounces whole wheat penne (or whole wheat pasta of your choice)^{GF}

1 cup (about 8 ounces) seeded and sliced cucumber

1 cup (about 5 ounces) cherry tomatoes, halved

½ small (2½ ounces) diced red onion

1 medium (6 ounces) red bell pepper, seeded and diced

1 medium (6 ounces) green bell pepper, seeded and diced

½ cup Kalamata olives, halved (about 20 olives)

½ cup crumbled feta cheese

Dressing

1 tablespoon Dijon mustard

¼ cup lemon juice

1 clove garlic, finely minced or grated

1 teaspoon dried oregano leaves

¼ teaspoon ground black pepper

⅓ cup olive oil

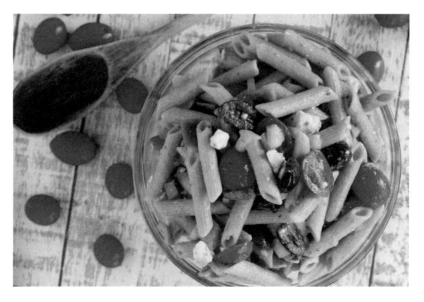

Prepare the pasta according to package directions. Drain and rinse under cool water to stop the cooking. Set aside.

To a large bowl, add the cooled pasta, cucumber, tomatoes, onion, bell peppers, olives, and feta cheese.

Whisk the mustard, lemon juice, garlic, oregano, and black pepper together in a small bowl. Pour in the olive oil while continuing to whisk. Blend until fully incorporated. Pour the dressing over the top of the pasta mixture and toss to coat. Cover and refrigerate at least 1 hour before serving.

Storage: Refrigerate in a sealed container for 3 to 4 days for best quality.

NUTRITION INFORMATION

PER SERVING: Calories 310; Fat 16g (Sat 3g); Protein 9g; Carb 35g; Fiber 8g; Calcium 86mg; Iron 3mg; Sodium 300mg; Folate 42mcg
ALLERGENS: Wheat, Milk
* = Gluten Free Option

FERTILITY FOCUS: Seeing a theme? Yep, whole grains and fiber-filled vegetables unite again in this delicious and nutritious combination. Plus, you get a hefty dose of antioxidants from the red and green bell peppers that complement those cherry tomatoes as they help rid your body of free radicals.

Italian Meatballs with Turkey and Mushrooms

 MAKES: 18 meatballs, 6 servings of 3 meatballs each
GLUTEN FREE*

Traditional beef meatballs get a makeover with a beautiful blend of mushrooms, herbs, and lean ground turkey. If you're feeling adventurous, we suggest trying the DIY Ranch Mix (page 108) in place of the dried parsley. The possibilities for customization are endless!

4 ounces white mushrooms, finely diced
1 small (6 ounces) onion, finely diced
2 cloves garlic, minced
1 pound lean ground turkey
1 tablespoon dried parsley

2 teaspoons Italian seasoning
½ teaspoon ground black pepper
½ teaspoon kosher salt
⅓ cup whole wheat bread crumbs^{GF}
1 large egg

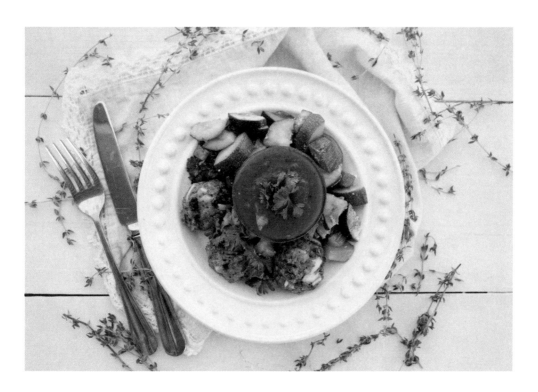

Preheat oven to 400°F. Line a large rimmed baking sheet with aluminum foil and spray with cooking spray.

Add mushrooms and onions to a large bowl and combine with minced garlic, ground turkey, parsley, Italian seasoning, black pepper, and salt. Mix thoroughly, then add breadcrumbs and egg. Continue to mix until incorporated.

Shape into 1-inch meatballs and space 1 inch apart on baking sheet. Bake 20 minutes, or until meatballs reach an internal temperature of 165°F.

Serve immediately alongside roasted vegetables or whole grain pasta or on a bed of tossed arugula, mixed greens, and olive oil.

Storage: Refrigerate in a sealed container for up to 4 days. Freeze for up to 3 months.

Shopping Tip: Whole wheat breadcrumbs can be purchased at most large markets in the specialty food aisle. If you can't find any, use two slices of whole grain bread, toast, and pulse into crumbs.

Kitchen Tip: To save time, place mushrooms in a food processor and pulse until finely chopped, about 20 seconds.

NUTRITION INFORMATION
PER SERVING: Calories 150; Fat 6g (Sat 1.5g); Protein 19g; Carb 7g; Fiber 1g; Calcium 18mg; Iron 1.1mg; Sodium 230mg; Folate 16mcg
ALLERGENS: Wheat, Egg
* = Gluten Free Option

FERTILITY FOCUS: Lean ground turkey is an excellent way to get heme iron (the most readily absorbed form of iron) in your diet while also satisfying those who enjoy animal protein every now and then. Plus, by blending with mushrooms, you also increase your intake of selenium and vitamin D—two other important nutrients that help support both male and female fertility.

Marinated Chicken Two Ways: Lemon Parsley and Cilantro Lime

MAKES: 4 servings, 4 ounces each
GLUTEN FREE

A simple marinade with plenty of flavor. Pair the Lemon Parsley Chicken with the Grecian Grain Bowl (page 208), or serve the Cilantro Lime Chicken on top of the Tex Mex Burrito Bowl (page 210) to deliver a hearty dose of lean protein.

1¼ pound boneless, skinless chicken
   breasts

Lemon Parsley Marinade
4 cloves garlic, chopped
¼ cup + 1 tablespoon olive oil
½ to ¾ cup Italian parsley, leaves and
   stems, washed (if milder flavor, use ½
   cup)
2 tablespoons water
¼ teaspoon ground black pepper
¼ teaspoon kosher salt
½ small lemon, thinly sliced

Cilantro Lime Marinade
4 cloves garlic, chopped
¼ cup + 1 tablespoon olive oil
1 cup cilantro, leaves and stems, washed
2 tablespoons water
¼ teaspoon cumin
¼ teaspoon ground black pepper
¼ teaspoon kosher salt
½ lime, thinly sliced

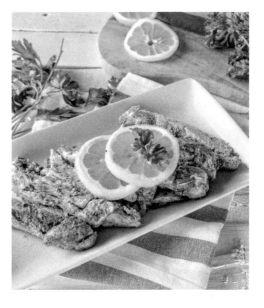

Place chicken breasts in a resealable plastic bag. Seal the bag and, using a meat mallet or rolling pin, pound the chicken until it is ½ inch thick.

    To prepare the marinade, combine the garlic, oil, herbs, water, spices, and salt in a blender or food processor and blend until smooth. Pour marinade and lemon slices into the bag with the chicken and seal the bag. Toss to coat. Remove any excess air from the bag and place chicken in the refrigerator to marinate. Marinate for at least 2 hours (up to 4 hours).

When ready to cook, remove chicken from the refrigerator. Place rack in the center of the oven and preheat oven to 375°F.

Use 1 tablespoon olive oil to coat the bottom of a 9 x 13-inch baking pan. Remove the chicken from the bag, discarding the marinade, and place the chicken in the pan and cover with foil.

Bake until chicken has reached an internal temperature of 165°F, about 20-25 minutes, flipping halfway through cooking time. Let rest before slicing.

Storage: Refrigerate in a sealed container for up to 4 days.

Kitchen Tip: Marinating chicken too long with acid can alter its texture. Allow ample time to prepare chicken prior to baking for best results.

NUTRITION INFORMATION

PER SERVING: Calories 170; Fat 5g (Sat 1g); Protein 29g; Carb 0g; Fiber 0g; Calcium 16mg; Iron 1.1mg; Sodium 80mg; Folate 6mcg

---

FERTILITY FOCUS: Traditional, store-bought marinades can be high in sodium. Too much sodium in your diet can lead to high blood pressure. Limiting dietary sodium by using fresh herbs adds flavor, reduces sodium intake, and helps make your body the healthiest it can be!

Slow Cooker Pulled Chicken

 MAKES: 10 servings, ½ cup
GLUTEN FREE

We're making your weeknights easy with this Slow Cooker Pulled Chicken. It makes a great base for tacos, sandwiches, salads—literally anything!

1 yellow onion, sliced (about 8 ounces)

1¼ pounds boneless, skinless chicken breasts

1 pound boneless, skinless chicken thighs

2 cloves garlic, smashed

1 bay leaf

¼ teaspoon ground black pepper

¼ teaspoon kosher salt

2 cups low sodium chicken broth

Place the onion in the bottom of a slow cooker. Top with chicken and add garlic, bay leaf, black pepper, and salt. Pour the broth over everything and cover the cooker with the lid. Cook on high for 4 hours or, preferably, on low for 8 hours.

Remove the chicken from the crock pot and transfer to a cutting board. Using two forks, carefully shred chicken.

To serve, toss chicken with BBQ sauce or a light vinaigrette and use as a filling for sandwiches. Alternatively, stuff into tortillas for tacos or burritos, or use as a topper for salads or other bowl dishes.

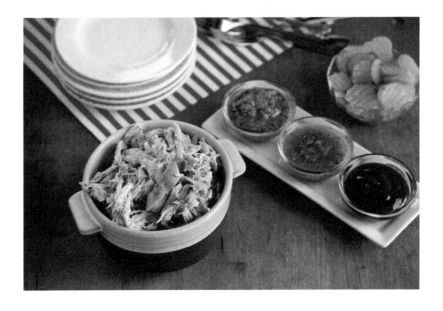

Storage: Refrigerate in a sealed container for up to 4 days, and freeze for up to 6 months.

Shopping Tip: Make friends with your local market's butcher. They will help guide you to finding the boneless, skinless chicken thighs in your store. They can also de-bone and skin them for you!

Kitchen Tip: Chicken breasts can be used in place of chicken thighs.

NUTRITION INFORMATION
PER SERVING: Calories 150; Fat 6g (Sat 1.5g); Protein 19g; Carb 7g; Fiber 2g; Calcium 54mg; Iron 3.3mg; Sodium 210mg; Folate 17mcg

FERTILITY FOCUS: Just like the Italian Meatballs, this is an excellent way to get heme iron in your diet. Iron is essential for brain development and plays a pivotal role in immunity. Though you can get iron from plant-based sources, our bodies most readily absorb this nutrient from animal sources.

Baked Mediterranean Chicken

MAKES: 4 servings of 1 chicken breast each
GLUTEN FREE

Looking for a simple, yet flavorful dish for dinner? This Baked Mediterranean Chicken comes together quickly and tastes great paired alongside the Greek Pasta Salad (page 190).

1 can (12 ounces) no salt added
    diced tomatoes, liquids and solids
2 cloves garlic, chopped
1 teaspoon dried oregano
⅓ rounded cup Kalamata olives,
    chopped (about 16 olives)
4 boneless, skinless chicken breasts
    (1¼ pound)
¼ cup crumbled feta cheese

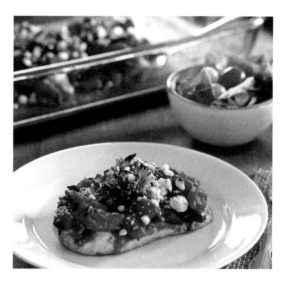

NUTRITION INFORMATION
PER SERVING: Calories 210; Fat 9g (Sat 2g);
Protein 27g; Carb 6g; Fiber 1g; Calcium 78mg;
Iron 1mg; Sodium 650mg; Folate 11mcg
ALLERGENS: Milk

Preheat the oven to 400°F. Combine diced tomatoes, garlic, oregano, and olives in a mixing bowl and set aside.

Coat a 9 x 13-inch glass baking dish with nonstick cooking spray. Place chicken breasts evenly in the bottom of the baking dish. Spoon the tomato mixture evenly over the chicken breasts, then sprinkle with feta cheese.

Bake in preheated oven for 30 to 35 minutes, or until chicken is cooked through and internal temperature reaches 165°F. Serve immediately.

Storage: Refrigerate in a sealed container for up to 4 days.

FERTILITY FOCUS: Canned tomatoes fill this baked chicken dish with heart-healthy antioxidants. Antioxidants are a great addition to a fertility-fueling diet that helps to rid the body of free radicals that can disrupt ovulation and lead to hormone imbalance.

PIZZA

Think you can't make your own pizza dough? Think again! We've got two hearty, healthy, and amazingly delicious dough recipes. If you've got some extra time, whip up the Taste of Italy Pizza Dough and find out just how our secret ingredient (bread flour) creates the perfect chewy pizza crust! Tight on time? No worries, the Quick Pizza Dough will be your new best friend!

FERTILITY FOCUS: Can you guess which ingredient has the starring role? Bingo, whole wheat flour! You can still enjoy a delicious pizza on your fertility journey by thinking ahead and preparing one of these nutrient-dense doughs. Whole grains help stabilize your blood sugars, which is crucial to achieving a fertile environment.

Taste of Italy Pizza Dough

MAKES: 2 dough balls of 16 ounces each (two 12-inch pizzas)
VEGETARIAN

1 package active dry yeast
   (or 2¼ teaspoons)
⅓ cup + 1 cup warm water
   (100 to 110°F)
1 teaspoon granulated sugar
1½ cups bread flour

2 cups whole wheat flour or white
   whole wheat flour
1 tablespoon honey
¼ cup olive oil
1½ teaspoons kosher salt

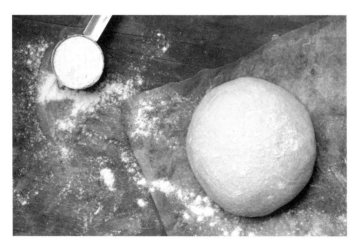

Place the yeast in a mixing bowl or in the bowl of a stand mixer. Add ⅓ cup of warm water and 1 teaspoon of sugar and let stand for about 8 to 10 minutes.

Add the flours, honey, olive oil, salt, and remaining water. Stir on low using the dough hook attachment (if using a stand mixer) until combined.

Turn the dough out on a floured work surface and knead until dough is elastic, about 4 minutes. If using a stand mixer, you can also turn it to a speed just above mixing and "knead" for about 5 to 6 minutes.

Shape dough into a ball, coat the bowl with nonstick cooking spray, and place the dough back in the bowl.

Cover with plastic wrap (spray the inside of the plastic wrap with nonstick cooking spray to prevent dough from sticking) and set in a warm, draft-free place for about 1 hour.

Uncover and punch down dough. Shape into 2 equal balls, placing the second ball in another coated bowl. Let rise another hour. Shape dough for pizza.

Storage: Cover and refrigerate overnight. When ready to use, remove from fridge and allow it to come to room temperature, or freeze for up to 2 months in tightly wrapped sealed container.

Kitchen Tip: Bread flour has more gluten, a protein found in wheat. The higher gluten content makes the dough more elastic (chewy), which works perfect for pizza!

Shopping Tip: Bread flour can be found in the baking aisle at most large markets. If unable to locate, substitute with all-purpose flour.

NUTRITION INFORMATION
PER SLICE: Calories 100; Fat 2.5g (Sat 0g); Protein 3g; Carb 15g; Fiber 2g; Calcium 2.1mg; Iron 0.8g; Sodium 120mg; Folate 13mcg
ALLERGENS: Wheat

Quick Pizza Dough

 MAKES: 1 dough ball of 16 ounces, (one 12-inch pizza)
VEGETARIAN

1 package active dry yeast (or 2¼
    teaspoons)
1 teaspoon granulated sugar
¾ to 1 cup warm water (125°F)
2 cups white whole wheat flour +
    extra for kneading
2 tablespoons olive oil
1 teaspoon kosher salt

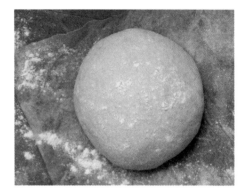

Add yeast and sugar to warm water in a large bowl. Let sit 10 minutes. Add the flour, olive oil, and salt, mixing with a wooden spoon for 3 to 5 minutes or until combined. Knead dough for about 5 minutes on a floured work surface. Remove from bowl.

Spray bowl with cooking spray and set dough back inside. Cover with plastic wrap and let rest in a warm place until doubled in size, about 1 hour.

When ready to make pizza, roll out dough on floured working surface and assemble as desired.

NUTRITION INFORMATION
PER SLICE: Calories 100; Fat 2.5g (Sat 0g); Protein 3g; Carb 15g; Fiber 3g; Calcium 1mg; Iron 0.8g; Sodium 160mg; Folate 2mcg
ALLERGENS: Wheat

Spinach and Sun-Dried Tomato Pizza

MAKES: One 12-inch pizza (12 slices, 2 slices per serving)
GLUTEN FREE*, VEGETARIAN

A veggie-based pizza is a perfect way to get dinner on the table fast. Serve it with a simple salad and our Italian Vinaigrette (page 161) to make it a complete meal.

16 ounces Quick Pizza Dough (page 201) or 1 pound refrigerated whole wheat pizza dough^{GF}

¼ cup Homemade Marinara Sauce (page 184) or store bought pizza sauce

2 cups (1½ ounces) fresh baby spinach

½ cup (1¾ ounces) thinly sliced red onion

½ cup (1¼ ounces) sun-dried tomatoes, chopped

1 cup shredded whole milk mozzarella cheese

¼ cup crumbled goat or feta cheese

1 teaspoon Italian seasoning

Coat a large bowl with nonstick cooking spray. Remove dough from packaging and place inside. Cover the top of the bowl with plastic wrap and rest on the counter to take the chill off, about 30 minutes.

Preheat the oven to 425°F and place the rack in the lowest shelf of the oven. (Don't skip this preheating step! It's important that your oven is warm before putting your pizza in there. If you have a pizza stone, use it.)

To make the pizza:

Dust your counter or other clean work surface lightly with flour (any flour will do). Remove dough from the bowl and place on your work surface. Using a rolling pin or your hands, shape dough into a 12-inch circle.

Transfer dough to a baking sheet or a pizza pan that has been coated with nonstick cooking spray or dusted with cornmeal. Spread marinara sauce over the crust and top with spinach, onions, sun-dried tomatoes, goat cheese, and mozzarella cheese. Sprinkle with Italian seasoning.

Transfer the pizza to the oven, sliding it directly onto a pizza stone, or leave it on an inverted cookie sheet before placing in the oven.

Bake for about 15 minutes, until cheese is melted and crust turns golden brown. Remove from oven, cut, and serve.

Variation: Feel free to use a variety of vegetables of your choice to create your own Veggie Supreme Pizza.

Storage: Refrigerate in a sealed container for up to 4 days. To reheat, turn oven to 350°F and bake on a baking sheet for 5 minutes.

NUTRITION INFORMATION
PER SERVING: Calories 310; Fat 12g (Sat 3.5g); Protein 12g; Carb 40g; Fiber 7g; Calcium 181mg; Iron 2.8mg; Sodium 590mg; Folate 83mcg
ALLERGENS: Wheat, Milk
* = Gluten Free Option

FERTILITY FOCUS: Have trouble fitting in vegetables? You're not alone! This pizza makes it easy to get plenty of the vegetables (which means plenty of the nutrients) your body needs for fueling fertility.

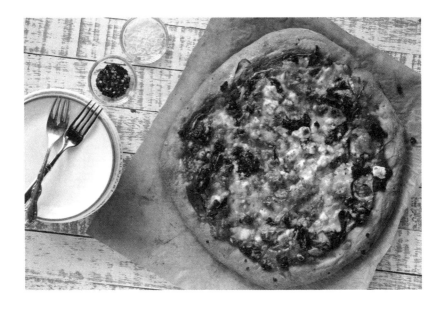

4-Layer Mexican Pizza
with Spicy Greek Yogurt Sauce

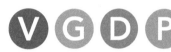

MAKES: 1 pizza, 12 slices each, 2 slices per serving
GLUTEN FREE*, VEGETARIAN

Nothing screams "fiesta!" like a Mexican Pizza. Serve this up as a party-pleasing food or for a simple Tuesday night dinner. There's no limit to when you can enjoy this fertility-fueling food.

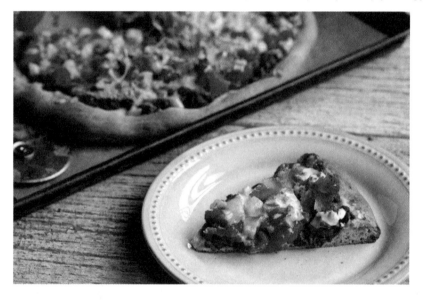

16 ounces Quick Pizza Dough
(page 201) or 1 pound refrigerated
whole wheat pizza dough^GF

1 can (15 ounces) no salt added black
beans, rinsed, and drained

1 can (14½ ounces) no salt added diced
tomatoes, divided

2 cloves garlic, minced

1½ teaspoons taco seasoning

½ medium (¾ cup, 4 ounces) red onion,
diced

1 medium (1½ cups, 6 ounces) green
bell pepper, diced

2 cups (6 ounces) shredded Mexican
cheese (or alternative cheese)

½ medium (3 ounces) avocado, diced,
for garnish

¼ cup fresh cilantro (optional garnish)

Spicy Yogurt Sauce

⅓ cup plain whole milk Greek yogurt

2 teaspoons rice vinegar

1 tablespoon water

1 teaspoon hot sauce

Preheat oven to 425°F and place rack in the lowest position. Coat a baking sheet or pizza pan with nonstick cooking spray or dust with cornmeal. Roll pizza dough out into a 12-inch circle and transfer to baking sheet.

Drain ½ cup of the diced tomato juice and place in a bowl with the taco seasoning. Discard the rest of the strained tomato juice and place diced tomatoes in a separate bowl. Mix with a fork to combine, then add the black beans and garlic and mash together using the back of a fork, about 3 to 5 minutes. Note: mixture will be slightly lumpy.

Spread the black bean mixture over the pizza dough as the sauce. Top with diced tomatoes, onions, and bell peppers. Sprinkle cheeses over the top and place in the oven. Cook for 18 to 20 minutes, or until cheese is melted and crust is crisp.

Remove and let sit 5 minutes before slicing.

Whisk the yogurt, rice vinegar, water, and hot sauce together. Top the pizza with diced avocados and cilantro, then drizzle the yogurt sauce over the pizza in a zigzag fashion. Cut into 12 slices.

Variation: If you do not have taco seasoning, use ½ teaspoon cumin, ½ teaspoon cayenne pepper, and ½ teaspoon paprika. Substitute any color bell pepper for the green bell pepper.

Storage: Refrigerate for up to 4 days. To reheat, turn oven to 350°F and bake on a baking sheet for 5 minutes.

NUTRITION INFORMATION

PER SERVING: Calories 410; Fat 15g (Sat 6g); Protein 19g; Carb 51g; Fiber 12g; Calcium 156mg; Iron 3.4mg; Sodium 620mg; Folate 94mcg

ALLERGENS: Wheat, Milk

* = Gluten Free Option

FERTILITY FOCUS: This pizza is a stellar, nutrient dense meal: filled with fiber from the beans, unsaturated fatty acids from the avocado and calcium from the cheese. Plus, you're getting a hefty dose of lycopene from the tomatoes! Remember, lycopene is an important nutrient linked to reproduction. Pizza for fertility? We say yes!

Sesame Tofu Stir Fry

MAKES: 4 cups, 4 servings
GLUTEN FREE, VEGAN

Busy nights call for easy recipes that satisfy. This stir fry is loaded with vegetarian protein and big flavor! Serve it over Sesame Noodles (page 240) to make it a complete dish!

14 ounces extra firm tofu (1 package)
1 tablespoon low sodium soy sauce
¼ cup low sodium vegetable broth
1 teaspoon cornstarch
1 tablespoon + 1 teaspoon canola oil
2 red, green or yellow bell peppers, diced (1¾ cup, 8½ ounces)
1 cup sliced carrot (5¼ ounces)
1 tablespoon fresh ginger, minced

1 clove garlic, minced
1 teaspoon sesame oil
1 tablespoon rice wine vinegar
1 tablespoon white or black sesame seeds
2 green onions, white and light green parts only, thinly sliced
Sriracha, as desired

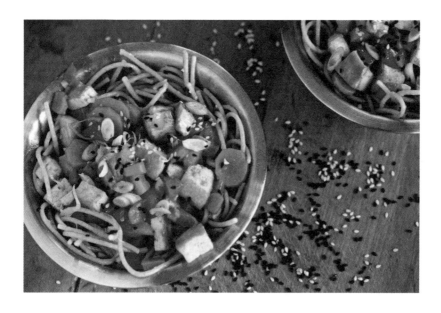

To prepare the tofu:

Remove tofu from the package and wrap tightly in a clean kitchen towel or several clean paper towels. Set on a plate and top with something heavy, such as a plate with a few cans stacked on top. Let sit for about 10 to 15 minutes. Remove tofu from towels and slice into ½-inch thick slices. Then cut slices into cubes.

To make the stir fry:

Mix the soy sauce, broth, and cornstarch together in a small bowl and set aside.

Set a wok or a large nonstick skillet over medium-high heat. Add 1 tablespoon canola oil and swirl around the skillet, then add the tofu and cook, stirring occasionally, until golden brown on all sides, about 8 to 10 minutes. Remove and reserve.

Add the remaining canola oil to the skillet, then add the bell pepper and carrot and cook 3 to 4 minutes. Stir in the ginger and garlic and cook 1 more minute, stirring often.

Stir the cornstarch mixture then and add to the skillet. Reduce heat to medium and cook until thickened, about 1 to 2 minutes. Turn off the heat and stir in the tofu, sesame oil, and rice wine vinegar. Garnish with sesame seeds and green onions. Serve with sriracha, if desired.

Storage: Cover and refrigerate for up to 5 days in a sealed container.

Kitchen Tip: Freeze any extra broth. Portion into an ice cube tray and place in freezer until frozen. Once frozen, put in a freezer bag, labeled and dated, for use at another time.

NUTRITION INFORMATION
PER SERVING: Calories 170; Fat 8g (Sat 1g); Protein 13g; Carb 11g; Fiber 3g; Calcium 208mg; Iron 2.9mg; Sodium 190mg; Folate 53mcg
ALLERGENS: Soy

FERTILITY FOCUS: Plant-based diets have proven to be extremely successful in promoting fertility (refer to page 11 in Chapter 2). This meal packs in over 10 grams of plant-based protein and is loaded with phytonutrients from the vegetables. Truly a winning combo to help achieve your most fertile self!

Grecian Grain Bowl

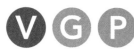

MAKES: 4 servings. 1 bowl each
GLUTEN FREE*, VEGETARIAN

Sneak away to the Mediterranean coast with this beautiful Grecian Couscous Grain Bowl! The wonderful flavors of fresh herbs and the rich, savory crumbled feta come together in this hearty, fiber-filled bowl.

2 cups cooked whole grain (whole wheat couscous)^{GF}

Feta Greek Yogurt Dressing

⅓ cup + 1 tablespoon plain whole milk Greek yogurt

2 tablespoons (1 ounce) crumbled feta cheese

1 tablespoon white wine vinegar

2 teaspoons water

¼ teaspoon garlic powder

⅛ teaspoon ground black pepper

⅛ teaspoon dried dill

⅛ teaspoon kosher salt

Bowl Assembly

2½ teaspoons olive oil, divided

1 teaspoon Italian seasoning

6 cups spring mix

2 cups ¼-inch diced tomatoes
   (or 2 cups cherry tomatoes, halved)

⅛ teaspoon kosher salt

1 can (15½ ounces) no salt added
   garbanzo beans, rinsed and drained

½ cup chopped roasted, unsalted
   pistachios

In a small bowl, combine yogurt, feta, vinegar, water, and spices. Mix thoroughly and set aside.

Mix cooled grains with 1 teaspoon of olive oil and Italian seasoning. In a separate bowl, combine the spring mix and chopped tomatoes with remaining olive oil and salt.

Portion salad among four serving dishes. Top with equal portions cooled grain, garbanzo beans, pistachios, and feta cheese. Serve with 2 tablespoons of Feta Greek Yogurt Dressing and toss to combine.

Storage: Refrigerate ingredients separately in sealed containers up to 5 days for maximum quality. Prepare bowl prior to eating or storing for lunch.

Kitchen Tip: Cook grain according to package instructions or refer to page 225 for whole grain cooking times.

NUTRITION INFORMATION

PER SERVING: Calories 230; Fat 9g (Sat 2g); Protein 11g; Carb 28g; Fiber 6g; Calcium 113mg; Iron 1.9mg; Sodium 260mg; Folate 35mcg

ALLERGENS: Wheat, Tree Nuts, Milk

* = Gluten Free Option

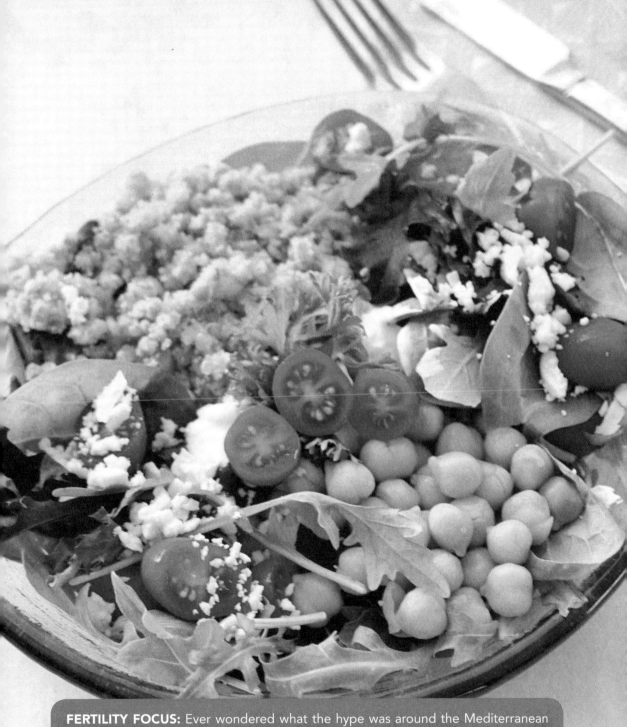

FERTILITY FOCUS: Ever wondered what the hype was around the Mediterranean diet? It's not just a fad; there's solid evidence that supports the health boosting properties of this way of eating, especially regarding fertility. The Mediterranean diet is centered on plant-based proteins like beans and legumes, whole grains, and heart-healthy fats like olive oil and nuts.

Tex Mex Burrito Bowl

MAKES: 4 servings, 1 bowl each
GLUTEN FREE, VEGETARIAN, VEGAN*

Savor the flavor of the Southwest from the comfort of your own home! Whip this up for a last-minute gathering and pair it with the Oven Baked Chips (page 112) and No Fail Guacamole (page 116) for a fun meal.

2 cups cooked whole grain (brown rice)
1 can (15 ounces) no salt added yellow corn kernel, rinsed and drained
1 can (15½ ounce) no salt added black beans, rinsed and drained
2 teaspoons olive oil, divided
1 teaspoon chili powder
½ teaspoon dried garlic powder
½ teaspoon smoked paprika
⅛ teaspoon kosher salt
1 jalapeños, seeded and chopped
2 hearts (6 cups) romaine lettuce, chopped

2 cups Pico De Gallo (page 114) or store bought tomato salsa
8 tablespoons No Fail Guacamole (page 116) or 4 ounces sliced avocado
4 tablespoons Creamy Chipotle Salad Dressing^{VG} (page 160) or alternative dressing
¼ cup (1 ounce) sharp cheddar cheese, shredded (optional garnish)^{VG}

To a medium bowl, add corn, black beans, 1 teaspoon of olive oil, chili powder, garlic powder, smoked paprika, and salt. Stir well. In a smaller bowl, mix chopped jalapeño and romaine together with remaining teaspoon of olive oil.

When ready to serve, assemble four bowls by placing ½ cup of cooked grain and lettuce mix topped with equal portions of corn and bean blend, Pico De Gallo, and guacamole. Garnish with a dollop of Chipotle Dressing and cheddar cheese.

Storage: Refrigerate ingredients separately in sealed containers up to 5 days for maximum quality. Prepare bowl prior to eating or storing for lunch.

Kitchen Tip: Prepare in mason jars for a quick grab and go meal. Place cooked rice on the bottom, layer with corn and bean blend, salsa, and dressing. Omit guacamole, since it will likely brown. Top with the lettuce and cheese. Shake vigorously prior to eating.

NUTRITION INFORMATION
PER SERVING: Calories 300; Fat 7g (Sat 2g); Protein 13g; Carb 49g; Fiber 13g; Calcium 162mg; Iron 4.3mg; Sodium410mg; Folate 356mg
ALLERGENS: Milk
* = Vegan Option ˚

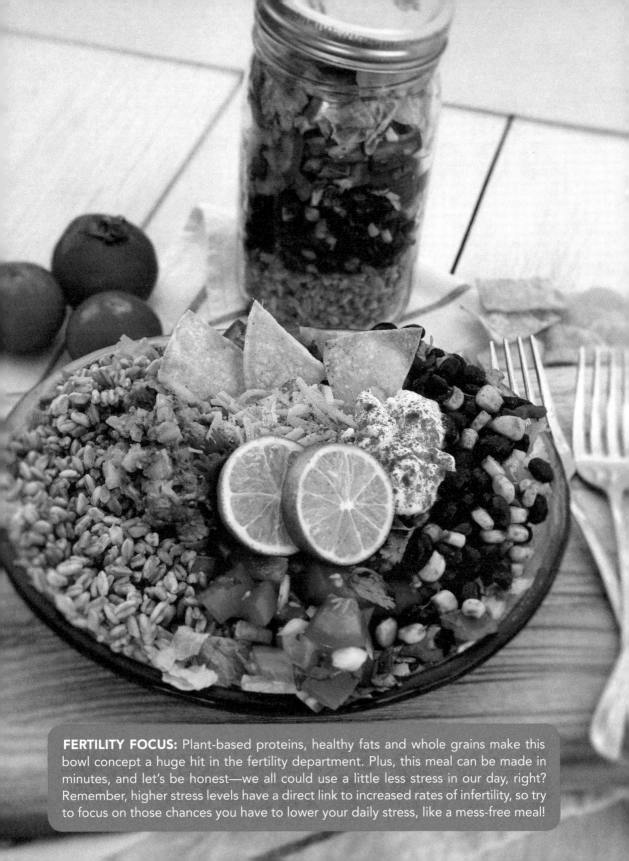

FERTILITY FOCUS: Plant-based proteins, healthy fats and whole grains make this bowl concept a huge hit in the fertility department. Plus, this meal can be made in minutes, and let's be honest—we all could use a little less stress in our day, right? Remember, higher stress levels have a direct link to increased rates of infertility, so try to focus on those chances you have to lower your daily stress, like a mess-free meal!

Protein Packed Freezer Burritos

MAKES: 12 servings of 1 burrito each
GLUTEN FREE*, VEGAN*

Don't buy burritos anymore! Make them yourself with delicious, nutritious ingredients to keep you satiated until your next meal.

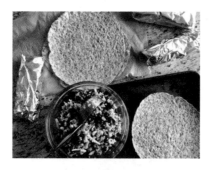

1 cup cooked quinoa
1 teaspoon ground cumin
1 teaspoon garlic powder
¼ teaspoon kosher salt
1 can (15 ounce) no salt added black beans, drained and rinsed
¾ cup frozen corn, thawed
½ cup tomatillo salsa
¾ cup shredded sharp cheddar cheese^VG
12 (8-inch) whole wheat or sprouted whole grain flour tortillas^GF

In a large mixing bowl, combine the quinoa, cumin, garlic powder, salt, black beans, corn, salsa, and cheddar cheese.

Lay tortillas out onto a clean work surface and spread ⅓ cup bean mixture down the middle of each tortilla.

To roll a burrito, fold one end of the tortilla to meet the other. Gently push back the tortilla and ingredients so that they are tight. Fold outside edges inward, then roll until burrito is closed. Roll in foil and repeat the process with the remaining burritos.

To serve, remove burritos from foil and place on a microwave-safe plate. Cover and cook on medium heat for about 4 to 6 minutes, turning once. Check and add more time if necessary. If you're unsure, use a food thermometer and cook until internal temperature reaches 165°F.

Variation: Top with plenty of nutritious ingredients. We love shredded lettuce, diced tomatoes, and onions, as well as guacamole and whatever your heart desires!

Storage: Refrigerate for up to 5 days. Freeze for up to 4 months.

Kitchen Tip: Freeze burritos in aluminum foil. Place a burrito in the center of each piece of foil and tightly roll up. Place foil-wrapped burritos in a freezer bag. Label and date them before freezing.

NUTRITION INFORMATION

PER SERVING: Calories 210; Fat 6g (Sat 2.5g); Protein 9g; Carb 30g; Fiber 6g; Calcium 150mg; Iron 1.9mg; Sodium 410mg; Folate 66mcg
ALLERGENS: Wheat, Milk
* = Vegan Option
* = Gluten Free Option

FERTILITY FOCUS: Whole grains and plant-based proteins combine in a convenient burrito to fuel your fertility. This dish helps your body maintain stable blood sugar while also delivering important B vitamins and high-quality protein. This is an excellent way to incorporate "fast food" into a fertility fueling meal plan. Plus, you can freeze these for later to help alleviate some of the stress that comes with the inevitable question, "What's for dinner?"

Stone-Ground Mustard and Apricot Glazed Salmon

MAKES: 2 servings, 3 ounces each
GLUTEN FREE

To ensure you are getting the most nutritious type of salmon, we recommend purchasing wild-caught salmon. Nutritionally speaking, wild caught fish is more nutrient-dense, has a better nutrition profile, and, in the case of salmon, has less saturated fat and more zinc, iron, and potassium than many other fish. If you're interested in trying another twist on using this superfood, we suggest the Smoked Salmon Breakfast Flatbread (page 70).

2, 4 ounce wild salmon fillets, with skin
1 tablespoon stone-ground mustard
2 teaspoons apricot preserves
¼ teaspoon kosher salt
Black pepper, freshly ground, to taste

NUTRITION INFORMATION
PER SERVING: Calories 200; Fat 8g (Sat 1.5g); Protein 26g; Carb 4g; Fiber 0g; Calcium 17mg; Iron 1.1mg; Sodium 380mg; Folate 29mcg
ALLERGENS: Fish

Preheat the broiler and place the oven rack about 5 to 6 inches away from the heat source. Line a rimmed cookie sheet or broiler pan with foil and coat with nonstick cooking spray.

In a small bowl, combine the mustard and apricot preserves.

Place the salmon on the prepared pan, skin side down. Sprinkle with salt and pepper. Place in the oven and broil for 5 minutes. Remove and spread mustard mixture evenly over the top and cook an additional 5 to 6 minutes, or until internal temperature reaches 145°F.

Storage: Cover and refrigerate in a sealed container for up to 3 days.

Kitchen Tip: Refer to the Monterey Bay Aquarium Seafood Watch to pick the most sustainable option.

Shopping Tip: Stone-ground mustard is also referred to as whole-grain mustard. You can find this in the condiment aisle. It is prepared using the whole mustard seed.

FERTILITY FOCUS: Salmon is, without question, an excellent addition to a fertility-fueled diet! It's packed with omega-3s, the heart-healthy fat that helps promote cardiovascular function, brain health, and improved mood. We know how moody this rollercoaster of fertility can make us, so we try to incorporate this entree at least weekly in our meal plan and encourage you to do the same!

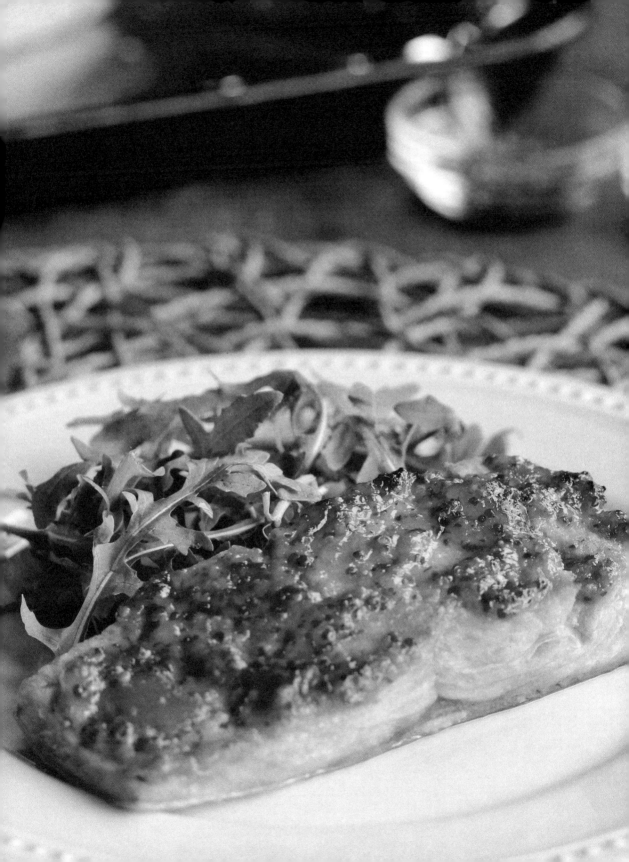

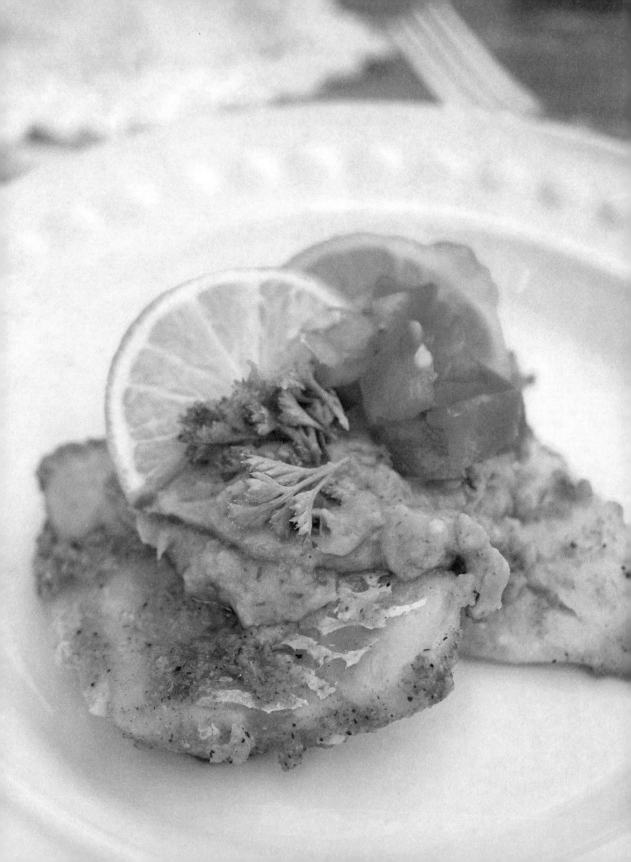

Pan-Seared Cod with Cumin and Avocado Cream

 MAKES: 4 servings of 4 ounces cooked fish each (makes a little over ½ cup sauce)
GLUTEN FREE*

½ small (3 ounces) avocado, peeled and seeded
2 tablespoons lime juice
¼ cup cilantro, roughly chopped
1 clove garlic
1 small jalapeño, roughly chopped (seeded if less spice is desired)
3 tablespoons water
⅛ teaspoon + ¼ teaspoon kosher salt
¼ teaspoon black pepper
1 teaspoon ground cumin
1¼ pounds cod fillets, skinned
2 tablespoons whole wheat flour (or finely ground cornmeal or masa flour)GF
1 tablespoon olive oil (or vegetable oil)
1 cup diced tomato
¼ cup diced red onion
Cilantro leaves, for garnish

In a blender or the bowl of a food processor, combine the avocado, lime juice, cilantro, garlic, jalapeño, water, and ⅛ teaspoon salt. Puree until smooth.

In a small bowl, combine ¼ teaspoon salt, black pepper and cumin. Pat the fish dry with clean paper towels and season both sides with the salt mixture, then dust with flour.

Set a large non-stick pan over medium-high heat and add the oil. Add the fish, skin side up, to the pan and cook, undisturbed for about 5 minutes. Turn fillets over and cook an additional 5 minutes, or until internal temperature reaches 145°F.

Transfer the fish to plates and serve with the avocado cream and garnish with the diced tomato, red onion and cilantro.

Variation: Other mild fish such as tilapia or whitefish will work here, too.

Storage: Refrigerate in a sealed container for up to 3 days.

NUTRITION INFORMATION
PER SERVING: Calories 180; Fat 7g (Sat 1g); Protein 23g; Carb 8g; Fiber 3g; Calcium 29mg; Iron 1mg; Sodium 620mg; Folate 37mcg
ALLERGENS: Wheat, Fish
* = Gluten Free Option

Blackened Shrimp

 MAKES: 4 servings, 3 ounces cooked shrimp
GLUTEN FREE

This Blackened Shrimp is the perfect weeknight dinner solution. Everything comes together quickly, so you'll have dinner on the table in no time.

1 teaspoon ground smoked paprika
1 teaspoon garlic powder
¼ teaspoon kosher salt
¼ teaspoon ground black pepper
1 teaspoon onion powder
¼ teaspoon cayenne pepper
1 teaspoon dried thyme leaves

1 pound large (31 to 40 count per pound) shrimp, peeled and deveined, with tails on
2 tablespoons olive oil
¼ cup fresh parsley, chopped
1 lemon, quartered

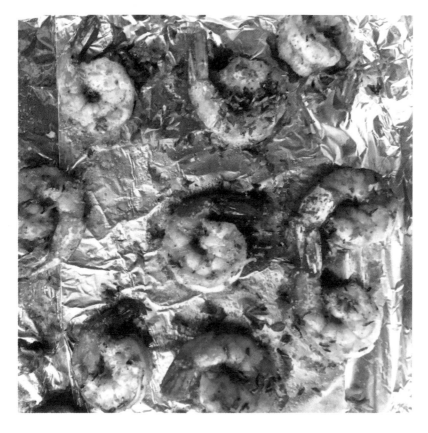

Preheat the oven to 375°F.

In a large bowl, combine the paprika, garlic powder, salt, pepper, onion powder, cayenne, and thyme. Add shrimp and oil and toss to coat. Pour shrimp out in an even layer onto a large rimmed baking sheet and cook shrimp about 8 to 10 minutes, or until internal temperature reaches 145°F.

Remove from the oven and toss with the parsley. Serve immediately with lemon wedges.

Storage: Refrigerate in a sealed container for up to 3 days.

Kitchen Tip: There are several sizes of shrimp, and labeling can be confusing. The numbers on the package represent how many shrimp you'll get per pound. For example, shrimp labeled "26/30" means you'll be getting 26 to 30 shrimp per pound. For less spice, reduce cayenne to ⅛ teaspoon.

NUTRITION INFORMATION
PER SERVING: Calories 150; Fat 8g (Sat 1.5g); Protein 16g; Carb 4g; Fiber 1g; Calcium 80mg; Iron 1.1mg; Sodium 770mg; Folate 30mcg
ALLERGENS: Shellfish

FERTILITY FOCUS: Shrimp provides not only lean protein, but also 100 percent of your Daily Value (or DV, see page 267) of selenium, a trace element and antioxidant that may help with sperm motility when combined with vitamin E. Plus, women need more selenium when breastfeeding, so why not prepare your body in advance?

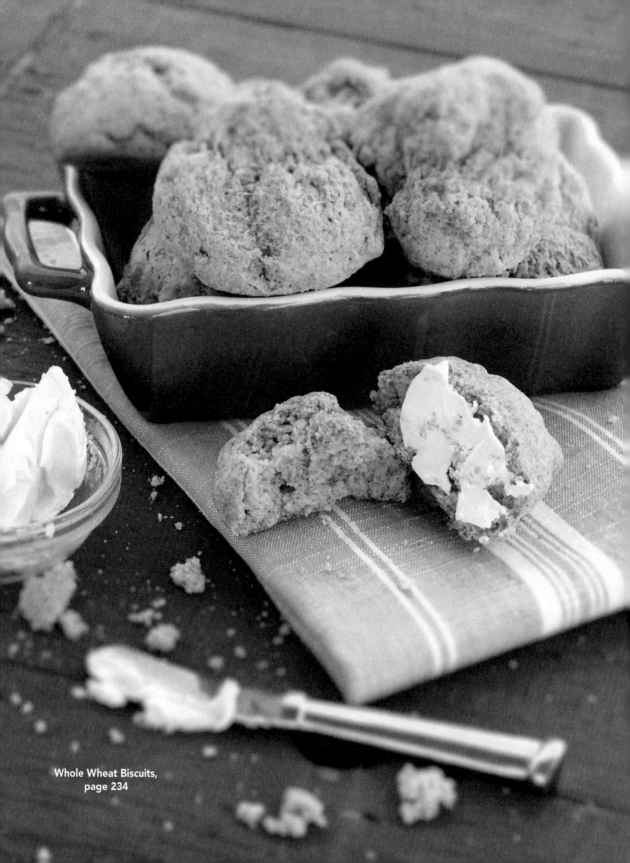

Whole Wheat Biscuits,
page 234

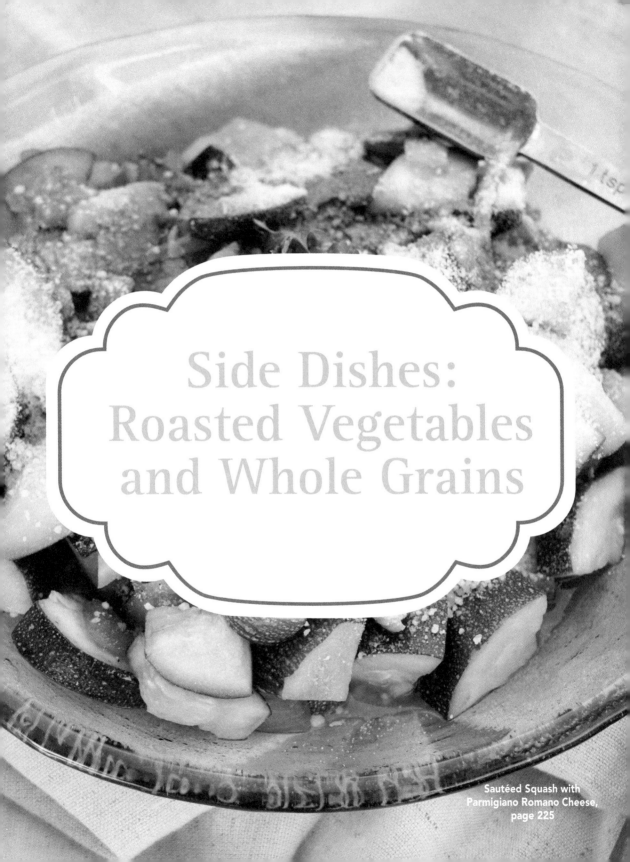

Side Dishes: Roasted Vegetables and Whole Grains

Sautéed Squash with
Parmigiano Romano Cheese,
page 225

W ONDERING WHAT TO PAIR with those entrees?
How about one of these nourishing sides?
As you know from our discussion in Chapter 2, we are *big* fans of the vegetable and whole grains food groups. The best thing about them is that there are countless ways to include them in your fertility-fueling diet. That's why we're providing some simple, basic recipes in this section, followed by a few variations to help inspire you in the kitchen.

ROASTED AND SAUTÉED VEGETABLES

General Info: Wash all produce before preparing. Cut all vegetables to about the same size for more even cooking. Refer to page 274 for knife cuts.

Servings: All recipes in the vegetable chart will yield 4 servings (about ½ cup each).

To Roast: Preheat oven to 425°F while prepping vegetables. Toss vegetables in 1 tablespoon olive oil, ¼ teaspoon kosher salt, and ¼ teaspoon black pepper, and then spread out onto a large, rimmed baking sheet. Roast according to chart.

To Sauté: Set a large sauté pan or skillet over medium-high heat. Once hot, add 1 tablespoon oil and swirl the pan to coat the bottom with oil. Add the vegetable, ¼ teaspoon kosher salt, and ¼ teaspoon black pepper. Refer to chart for cooking time.

To Blanch and Shock: Fill a large bowl with water and ice and set aside. Set a large pot filled with about 4 quarts of water over high heat, add 2 tablespoons kosher salt, and bring to a boil. Yes, 2 tablespoons of salt! (And no, we're not kidding. The salt seasons the food while providing a beautiful, vibrant color to the vegetables. Rest assured; most of the salt actually remains in the blanching liquid and does not significantly increase the total sodium of the dish.) Add vegetables, stir, and blanch according to chart. Strain vegetable from boiling water and place in ice water to stop the cooking process.

To Finish: During the last few minutes of cooking, add dried herbs such as oregano, Italian seasoning, rosemary, or thyme. Or, at the end of cooking, add chopped fresh herbs such as basil, chives, parsley, dill, rosemary, cilantro, tarragon, or basil. Stir in toasted nuts or seeds. Add a drizzle of balsamic vinegar, red wine vinegar, or champagne vinegar, or a splash of lime or lemon juice. Or, cook up some garlic to toss in at the end.

Vegetable (fresh)	How to Prep	Roasting Method	Sauté Method
Asparagus (1 pound, or about 1 bunch)	Trim bottom parts of stalks. Leave whole or cut into thirds.	Roast, stirring once, for 12 to 15 minutes.	Blanch about 1 minute and shock. Sauté, stirring frequently, about 5 to 8 minutes.
Bell Peppers (1¼ pound)	Core and stem peppers, then cut into 1-inch slices.	Roast, stirring once, for 20 to 25 minutes.	Sauté, stirring frequently, about 10 minutes.
Broccoli (1 pound)	Trim off leaves then cut head into bite-size florets. Peel away the outer woody-part of the stem and then slice.	Roast, stirring once, for 15 to 20 minutes.	Blanch about 2 to 3 minutes and shock. Sauté, stirring frequently, about 4 to 6 minutes.
Brussels sprouts (1 pound)	Remove outer leaves and trim. Cut larger sprouts in half or quarter.	Roast, stirring once, for 15 to 20 minutes.	Blanch about 2 to 3 minutes and shock. Sauté, stirring frequently, about 3 to 5 minutes.
Carrots or Parsnips (1 pound)	Peel and trim. Slice into ½-inch pieces.	Roast, stirring once, for 20 minutes.	Sauté, stirring frequently, about 10 to 12 minutes.
Cauliflower (1 pound + 4 ounces)	Remove leaves and stem. Cut cauliflower into bite-size pieces.	Roast, stirring twice, for 30 to 40 minutes.	Blanch about 2 to 3 minutes and shock. Sauté, stirring frequently, about 2 to 4 minutes.
Green Beans (12 ounces)	Trimmed	Roast, stirring once, for 15 to 20 minutes.	Blanch about 3 minutes then shock. Sauté, stirring frequently, about 2 to 3 minutes.
Onions (1 pound + 2 ounces)	Cut into ⅛-inch slices	Roast, stirring twice, for 30 to 45 minutes.	Sauté, stirring frequently, about 10 to 12 minutes.
Potatoes, Sweet (1 pound + 4 ounces)	Peel and cut into large dice.	Roast, stirring twice, for 45 to 55 minutes.	Not preferred or par-boil then sauté, stirring frequently, about 10 to 12 minutes.
Potatoes, Yukon Gold (1 pound + 4 ounces)	Peel and cut into large dice.	Roast, stirring once or twice, for 25 to 30 minutes.	Not preferred or par-boil then sauté, stirring frequently, about 10 to 12 minutes.
Summer Squash, yellow and zucchini (1 pound)	Trim stem end. Cut into ½-inch slices or into a large dice.	Roast, stirring once, for 10 to 12 minutes.	Sauté, stirring frequently, about 10 to 12 minutes.

WHOLE GRAINS

General Info: Salt can be adding to cooking water, or grain can be seasoned to taste with kosher salt and black or white pepper after cooking.

Whole Grain	Grain to Liquid Ratio (in cups)	Cook Time
Quinoa*	1:2	12 to 15 minutes
Bulgur	1:2	15 to 20 minutes
Amaranth	1:3	20 minutes
Farro*	1: 2 ½	30 minutes
Wild Rice	1:3	35 to 45 minutes
Short Grain Brown Rice	1:2 ½	35 to 40 minutes
Long Grain Brown Rice	1:3	40 minutes
Millet	1:2	30 to 35 minutes
Whole-wheat couscous	1 to 1 ½ :1	5 minutes

Should be rinsed first

Sautéed Squash with Parmigiano Romano Cheese

 MAKES: 2 cups (4 servings of ½ cup each)
GLUTEN FREE, VEGETARIAN, VEGAN*

Squash is a vegetable that is easily lovable. Pair it with Parmigiano Romano cheese and you've got the perfect side for almost any meal.

2 medium (1 pound) zucchini, trimmed
1 tablespoon olive oil
½ small onion (2 ounces), roughly
    chopped
2 cloves garlic, minced
¼ teaspoon ground black pepper
⅛ teaspoon kosher salt
2 tablespoons grated Parmesan
    Romano cheese^{VG}
1 tablespoon balsamic vinegar

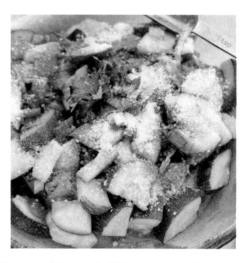

NUTRITION INFORMATION
PER SERVING: Calories 80; Fat 5g (Sat 1.5g); Protein 3g; Carb 6g; Fiber 1g; Calcium 69mg; Iron 0.5mg; Sodium 130mg; Folate 28mcg
ALLERGENS: Milk
* = Vegan Option Available

Slice zucchini in half lengthwise, then cut into ¼-inch slices.

Heat oil in a medium sauté pan over medium heat. Add onion and cook 3 minutes, stirring frequently. Place zucchini in the pan and cook on high heat for 6 to 7 minutes, or until fork tender.

Add garlic, pepper, and salt to the pan and cook another 2 to 3 minutes. Remove from heat and garnish with Parmesan Romano cheese. Serve hot and garnish with balsamic vinegar. Best if eaten immediately.

Storage: Place in a sealed container, refrigerate and consume within 1 day.

FERTILITY FOCUS: We are firm believers that plants are a key component in a fertility fueling diet. Not only do plants like zucchini provide a great source of nutrients, but they also pair wonderfully over a simple whole grain, like quinoa, to provide a complete plant-based meal.

Roasted Cauliflower with Chipotle Cream

MAKES: 4 servings, ½ cup each
GLUTEN FREE, VEGETARIAN

Cauliflower gets a makeover in this delicious and nutritious dish! The chipotle cream is the perfect complement to the fiber-filled white goddess.

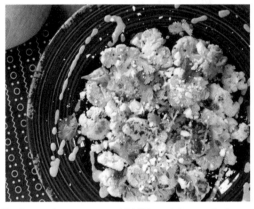

1 cauliflower head, trimmed and cut
   into ¼-inch slices
2 tablespoons olive oil
¼ teaspoon kosher salt
¼ teaspoon ground black pepper
½ teaspoon ground chipotle powder
   (or ½ teaspoon chipotle paste)
¼ cup plain whole milk Greek yogurt
2 tablespoons lemon juice
1 clove garlic, grated or minced
1 teaspoon honey
¼ cup crumbled feta cheese
¼ cup chopped cilantro

NUTRITION INFORMATION

PER SERVING: Calories 140; Fat 10g (Sat 3g); Protein 6g; Carb 11g; Fiber 3g; Calcium 98mg; Iron 0.8mg; Sodium 260mg; Folate 88mcg
ALLERGENS: Milk

Preheat the oven to 400°F and line a baking sheet with foil. Place the sliced cauliflower onto the pan, drizzle both sides with olive oil, and season with salt and pepper. Place in the oven and bake for 20 to 25 minutes, turning once.

While cauliflower is cooking, make the Chipotle Cream Dressing. In a small bowl, whisk together the chipotle powder, Greek yogurt, lemon juice, garlic, and honey. Set aside.

Remove cauliflower from the oven and transfer to a serving dish. Drizzle some of the dressing over the cauliflower, then garnish with feta cheese and cilantro. Serve extra dressing on the side. Enjoy immediately.

Variation: Use chili powder in place of chipotle powder.

Storage: Place in a sealed container, refrigerate and consume within 1 day.

FERTILITY FOCUS: Filled with vitamin C, an important antioxidant, cauliflower is a great addition to your fertility-fueling diet. Antioxidants play a crucial role in helping rid your body of free radicals, which may be a cause of ovulatory infertility.

Garlic Spinach with Sliced Almonds

MAKES: 4 servings,
½ cup each
GLUTEN FREE, VEGAN

You know what pairs beautifully with spinach? Almonds and garlic! That's right, and it tastes great on top of the Parmesan Portobello Burger (page 126) or served with the Stone Ground Mustard and Apricot Glazed Salmon (page 214).

2 teaspoons olive oil
2 tablespoons sliced, unsalted almonds
1 clove garlic, minced
5 cups (5 ounces) baby spinach
⅛ teaspoon kosher salt
⅛ teaspoon ground black pepper

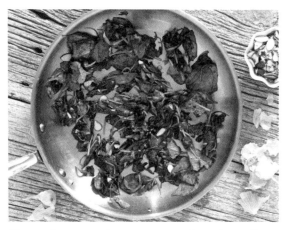

Heat a large sauté pan over medium heat. Once hot, add olive oil and almonds and cook, stirring frequently, for 1 minute. Add the garlic and cook an additional minute, stirring so as to not burn the garlic.

Add the spinach and toss gently, cooking until spinach is just wilted, about 2 to 3 minutes, adjusting heat if necessary. Take off the heat, garnish with salt and pepper, and serve immediately.

Storage: Place in a sealed container, refrigerate, and consume within 1 day.

NUTRITION INFORMATION
PER SERVING: Calories 50; Fat 3.5g (Sat 0g); Protein 2g; Carb 3g; Fiber 2g; Calcium 76mg; Iron 2.4mg; Sodium 115mg; Folate 135mcg
ALLERGENS: Tree nuts

FERTILITY FOCUS: Spinach contains plenty of vitamin A, calcium, and iron, and when you cook it, you absorb even more. Vitamin A helps with vision; calcium helps build and maintain bones; and iron is important in transporting oxygen throughout your body's cells. Phew! See now why spinach is so amazing?

Oven Baked French Fries

 MAKES: 4 servings, 3½ ounces per serving
GLUTEN FREE, VEGAN

Satisfy your craving for a "fried" crispy potato without the added fat, calories, and sodium typically found in fast food varieties. Serve a side of these spuds with our yummy Umami Burger (page 128).

1 large (14 ounces) russet potato, skin on, washed and cleaned
¾ teaspoon ground garlic powder
¾ teaspoon dried parsley
¼ teaspoon ground onion powder
¼ teaspoon ground black pepper
¼ teaspoon kosher salt
1 tablespoon olive oil
Fresh parsley, garnish

Preheat oven to 400°F. Line a baking sheet with parchment paper. Slice potatoes lengthwise into ¼-inch strips. In a small bowl, combine garlic, parsley, onion, pepper, and salt.

In a large bowl, toss sliced potatoes with olive oil. Sprinkle on spices and toss again. Spread potatoes out in an even layer on prepared pan. Bake for 18 minutes and flip with a spatula. Bake another 12 to 14 minutes, until potatoes are browned and crispy. Remove and serve immediately with desired dipping sauce.

Variation: Use a variety of russet and sweet potatoes. Not only will this help to increase your intake of vitamin A, an essential nutrient for reproduction, but also provide great flavor!

Storage: Place in a sealed container, refrigerate, and consume within 1 day.

NUTRITION INFORMATION
PER SERVING: Calories 140; Fat 7g (Sat 1g); Protein 2g; Carb 19g; Fiber 1g; Calcium 16mg; Iron 1mg; Sodium 125mg; Folate 15mcg

FERTILITY FOCUS: We've said it before, we'll say it again: do not deprive yourself! We know how satisfying a burger and fries combo can be, so we're providing a healthy option to enjoy it. While russet potatoes (also known as white potatoes) get a bad rap, it's important to point out they do provide important nutrients such as vitamin B6 and potassium.

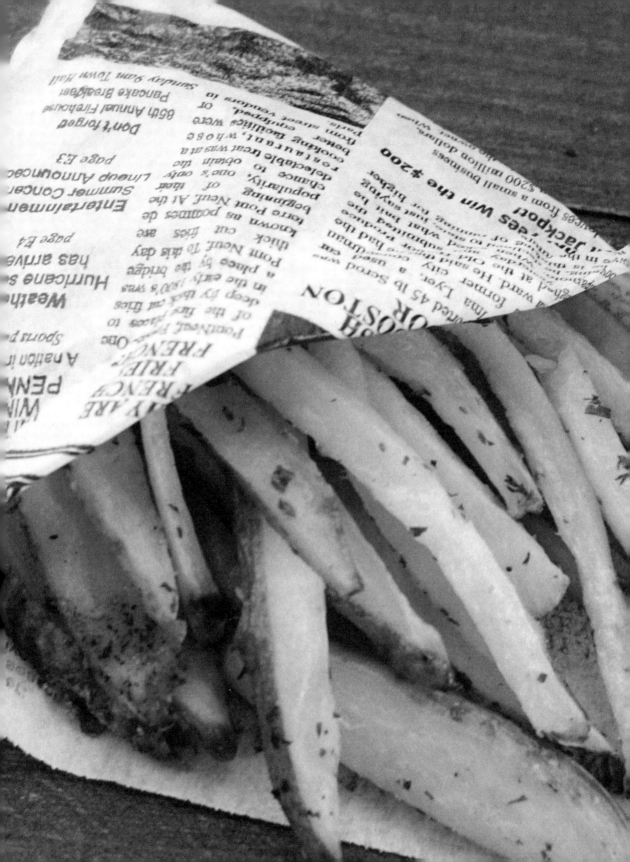

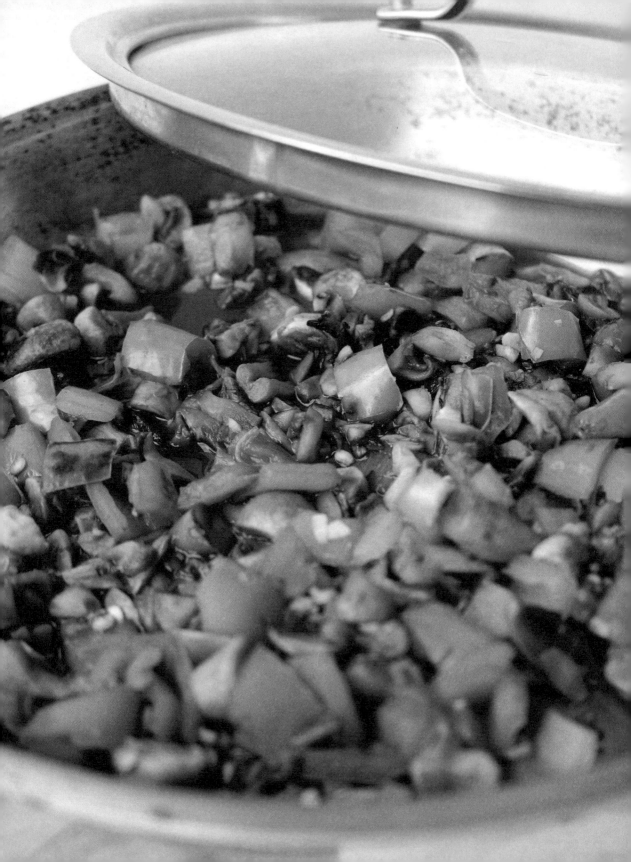

Sautéed Peppers and Mushrooms

MAKES: 2 cups (4 servings of ½ cup each)
GLUTEN FREE, VEGAN

Take your Umami Burger (page 128) up a notch by topping it with a little heat. These Sautéed Peppers and Mushrooms make the perfect condiment—they're low in sodium and fat, but high in flavor. You may just give your local burger joint a run for their money!

1 tablespoon olive oil

1 medium (7 ounces) green bell pepper, chopped

3 cups (8 ounces) white button mushrooms, sliced or chopped

2 medium (about 4 ounces) Serrano peppers, seeded and chopped (or jalapeno peppers)

2 tablespoons low sodium vegetable broth (or water)

3 cloves garlic, finely chopped

⅛ teaspoon of kosher salt

In a sauté pan over medium heat, add the olive oil, bell pepper, mushrooms, and Serrano peppers. Sauté for 3 to 5 minutes. Add the vegetable broth and garlic. Cook for additional 3 to 5 minutes until garlic is cooked. Remove from heat, add salt, and stir. Top your burger or salads or serve as a side.

Storage: Refrigerate in an airtight container or jar. Use within 2 days for optimum freshness.

NUTRITION INFORMATION

PER SERVING: Calories 60; Fat 3.5g (Sat 0g); Protein 2g; Carb 6g; Fiber 1g; Calcium 11mg; Iron 0.5mg; Sodium 125mg; Folate 14mcg

FERTILITY FOCUS: Condiments can be hidden sources of sodium and questionable preservatives. Instead of opting for the unknown, this simple recipe is loaded with science-backed fertility-fueling foods like mushrooms and olive oil. These ingredients combine beautifully to give your taste buds maximum satisfaction and your body 100% nutrient-dense food!

Pickled Cauliflower, Red Onions, and Jalapenos

MAKES: 8 servings, ¼ cup each
GLUTEN FREE, VEGAN

Move over, store-bought pickled jalapeños—we've got something that's sure to be your new favorite taco, salad, or sandwich topping!

½ medium red onion, sliced (about 1½ cups)

4 cups water

1 cup grated cauliflower

½ jalapeño, sliced

⅓ cup white wine vinegar

5 black peppercorns

2 tablespoons lime juice

⅓ cup orange juice

1 teaspoon kosher salt

Place the sliced onions in a medium, nonreactive bowl. Heat the water on the stove until boiling.

Once boiling, pour over onions. Let sit about 15 seconds, then strain the onions in a colander or sieve set over the sink. Once drained, transfer the onions back to the nonreactive bowl and add cauliflower and jalapeños. Set aside.

To the now-dry pot, add the vinegar, peppercorns, lime juice, orange juice, and salt. Set pot over medium heat and allow it to come to a boil, about 5 to 6 minutes.

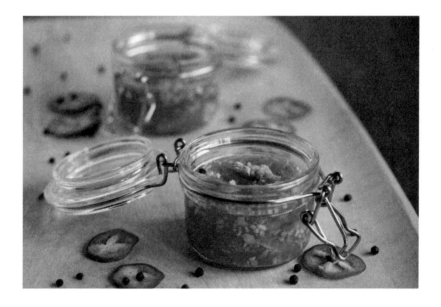

Remove from heat and pour over the onions. Stir, then pack mixture down with a spoon. Allow to cool about 20 to 30 minutes, then pack down again, cover, and refrigerate.

Let "pickle" in the fridge for at least 2 hours, though overnight is better. Remove from pickling liquid and enjoy!

Storage: Refrigerate in an airtight container or jar. Use within 7 days for best flavor.

Kitchen Tip: To make grated cauliflower (cauliflower rice), wash and pat dry a head of cauliflower. Remove the leaves and large stems and, using a box grater with medium grating holes or a food processor with the chopping attachment, grate/pulse cauliflower until it's the size of rice. One head of cauliflower will make about 4 cups of cauliflower rice.

NUTRITION INFORMATION
PER SERVING: Calories 20; Fat 0g (Sat 0g); Protein 1g; Carb 4g; Fiber 1g; Calcium 14mg; Iron 0.1mg; Sodium 70mg*; Folate 14mcg
* Sodium content calculated using approximate 25 percent absorption.

FERTILITY FOCUS: Filled with cauliflower, onions, and jalapeños, your body is getting a trifecta of flavor from this homemade condiment. Cauliflower is loaded with isothiocyanates, crucial phytonutrients that rid the body of potentially carcinogenic compounds. We can all agree, carcinogens are definitely not great for fertility!

Whole Wheat Biscuits

MAKES: 10 drop biscuits, 1 biscuit each
GLUTEN FREE*, VEGETARIAN

Nix the refrigerated tub of dough and whip up these simple, hearty biscuits. Filled with heart-healthy fats and a hefty dose of whole grains, you can freeze them to enjoy on the fly, for breakfast with the All Natural Berry Jam (page 57).

2 cups lightly scooped whole wheat
    white flour^{GF}
1 tablespoon baking powder
2 tablespoons dried thyme leaves
    (optional)
¾ teaspoon kosher salt
1 cup whole milk
¼ cup vegetable oil

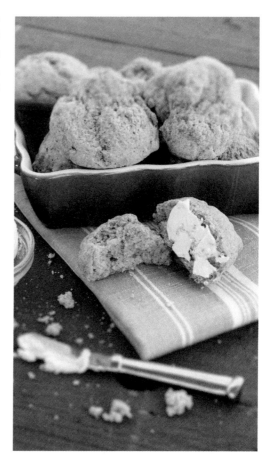

NUTRITION INFORMATION
PER SERVING: Calories 160; Fat 7g (Sat 1g);
Protein 4g; Carb 21g; Fiber 3g; Calcium 109mg;
Iron 1mg; Sodium 300mg; Folate 1mcg
ALLERGENS: Wheat, Milk
* = Gluten Free Option

Preheat oven to 400°F. In a large mixing bowl, whisk together the flour, baking powder, thyme, and salt.

In a separate bowl, add milk and oil, then add all at once to the dry ingredients. Stir to combine, mixing gently yet quickly, about 20 seconds.

On a greased baking sheet, drop 10 rounded spoonfuls of dough. Bake 20 to 22 minutes, until biscuit tops are golden brown. Remove from oven and let cool on a wire rack.

Variation: Many herbs work well here, so feel free to substitute rosemary, sage, fennel, or other favorites for the thyme. Or, if you prefer a traditional biscuit, forgo the addition of the herb altogether.

Storage: Store in a zip-top bag in the refrigerator for up to 1 week or freeze for up to 2 months.

Kitchen Tip: Whole wheat white flour is considered a 100% whole grain. The difference is it's made from white whole wheat, not the hard red spring wheat used in standard whole wheat. It's less grainy and dense, making it a great option in a light and flaky product like a biscuit.

FERTILITY FOCUS: Whole grains are essential for your fertility, so it's important to focus on fueling your body with as many sources of whole grains as possible. Not only will you help stabilize your blood sugar by eating grains that contain fiber and protein, but you'll also enjoy the delicious and nutritious joy of a warm and fresh biscuit!

Sautéed Mushrooms with Thyme and Bulgur

MAKES: 6 servings, ½ cup each
VEGAN

Finely chopped mushrooms, sautéed until golden, then tossed with bulgur, fresh thyme, and pine nuts. It's the perfect complement to the French Lentil Salad with Spinach and Feta (page 158); or make it a complete meal by topping it with Slow Cooker Pulled Chicken (page 196).

¾ cup bulgur
¼ + ⅛ teaspoon kosher salt
1½ cups boiling water
2 tablespoons pine nuts
1 teaspoon olive oil 1 tablespoon olive oil
2 tablespoons finely chopped shallot

8 ounces mushrooms (cremini or a blend), cleaned and chopped
1 clove garlic, chopped
⅛ teaspoon black pepper
1 teaspoon fresh thyme leaves, chopped

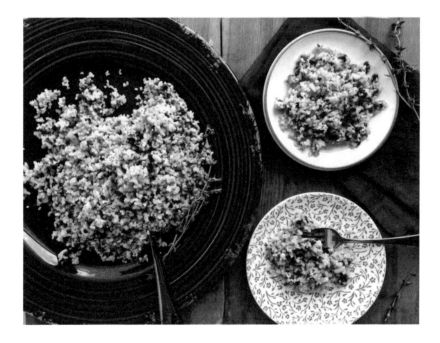

Place bulgur in a medium bowl. Add ¼ teaspoon salt, then cover with boiling water. Immediately cover the bowl with a piece of plastic wrap and let bulgur steam for about 20 minutes.

Heat a skillet over medium-high heat. Add the pine nuts and toast, stirring occasionally, until lightly browned, about 3 to 4 minutes. Remove from pan and reserve.

Turn heat down to medium and add the olive oil to the skillet. Add the shallot and sauté until softened, about 2 to 3 minutes. Increase heat to medium-high, add the chopped mushrooms and ⅛ teaspoon of salt, and cook another 5 minutes.

Remove plastic wrap from the bulgur and drain any excess liquid. Add the mushroom mixture, toasted pine nuts, black pepper, and fresh thyme to the bulgur; stir to combine. Garnish with extra thyme, if desired, and serve.

Storage: Refrigerate for up to 5 days in an airtight container.

Kitchen Tip: Fresh thyme can be substituted with a rounded ¼ teaspoon dried thyme leaves.

NUTRITION INFORMATION
PER SERVING: Calories 110; Fat 5g (Sat 0.5g); Protein 3g; Carb 16g; Fiber 3g; Calcium 18mg; Iron 0.7mg; Sodium 130mg; Folate 17mcg
ALLERGENS: Wheat, Tree Nuts

FERTILITY FOCUS: Mushrooms and bulgur are a great combo for powering your fertility! Mushrooms are filled with vitamin D (an important nutrient for your fertility), and bulgur is a whole grain, supplying fiber and other powerful fertility-friendly nutrients. When paired with fresh herbs and spices, this duo creates a delicious and nutritious addition to your fertility-fueling diet.

Turmeric Wild Rice Pilaf

  **MAKES: 3 cups,
6 servings, ½ cup each**
GLUTEN FREE, VEGAN

Join the trend and get on the turmeric train! We've taken this super spice and incorporated it into a traditional rice pilaf to provide your body with total nourishment. It tastes wonderful with the Lemon Parsley Marinated Chicken (page 194).

2½ cups water
1 cup wild rice, rinsed
½ teaspoon kosher salt, divided
1 tablespoon olive oil
1 small (3½ ounces) onion, chopped
2 medium (3 ounces) carrots, peeled and chopped
1 (1½ ounces) celery stalk, chopped
2 cloves garlic, minced
1 cup low sodium vegetable broth
1 cup green peas (or frozen mixed vegetable blend)
1 tablespoon ground turmeric
¾ teaspoon ground smoked paprika
½ teaspoon ground black pepper
¼ cup fresh cilantro, chopped (optional garnish)

Boil water in a medium saucepot, then add rice and ¼ teaspoon salt. Reduce heat to simmer and cover, cooking until rice is just tender, about 30 to 35 minutes. Remove from heat and drain.

Heat oil in a large skillet over medium heat. Add onion, carrots, and celery, and cook for 5 minutes, until softened. Add garlic and cook 5 minutes.

Add the rice and stir in vegetable broth, peas (or frozen vegetables), turmeric, paprika, black pepper, and the remaining ¼ teaspoon salt. Cook over medium heat until broth is absorbed, approximately 5 to 8 minutes. Garnish with fresh cilantro and serve.

Shopping Tip: You can find ground turmeric in the spice aisle.

Storage: Refrigerate for up to 5 days in an airtight container.

NUTRITION INFORMATION
PER SERVING: Calories 160; Fat 3.5g (Sat 0g); Protein 4g; Carb 31g; Fiber 4g; Calcium 20mg; Iron 1.3mg; Sodium 190mg; Folate 18mcg

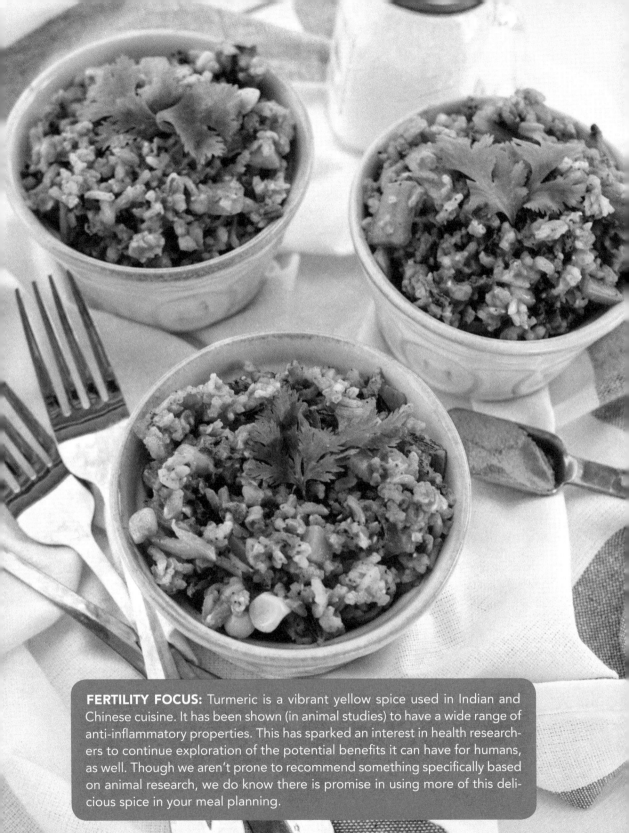

FERTILITY FOCUS: Turmeric is a vibrant yellow spice used in Indian and Chinese cuisine. It has been shown (in animal studies) to have a wide range of anti-inflammatory properties. This has sparked an interest in health researchers to continue exploration of the potential benefits it can have for humans, as well. Though we aren't prone to recommend something specifically based on animal research, we do know there is promise in using more of this delicious spice in your meal planning.

Sesame Noodles

MAKES: 5 servings, 1 cup each
GLUTEN FREE*, VEGAN

These sesame noodles are perfect to pair with our Sesame Tofu Stir Fry (page 206) or top with cooked shrimp, chicken, or edamame!

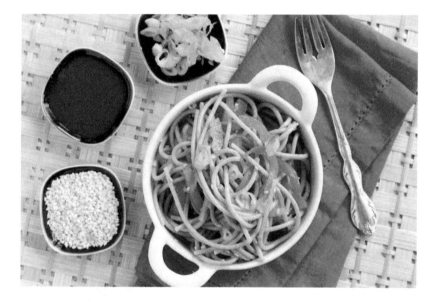

8 ounces whole wheat spaghetti^{GF}

2 tablespoons canola oil

1 tablespoon sesame oil

2 cloves garlic, minced

1 tablespoon fresh ginger, minced

¼ teaspoon kosher salt

1 tablespoon + 2 teaspoons rice wine vinegar

1 teaspoon low sodium soy sauce^{GF}

3 green onions, white and light green parts only, thinly sliced

1 red bell pepper (5 ½ ounces), thinly sliced (about 1½ cups sliced)

1 teaspoon sesame seeds (white or black)

Sriracha, to taste

Prepare the noodles according to package directions. Drain and rinse under cold water until cool to the touch, removing any excess water. Set aside.

In a large mixing bowl, whisk together the oils, garlic, ginger, salt, vinegar, and soy sauce. Stir in the green onions, bell pepper, and sesame seeds. Add the cooked noodles and toss until well coated. Garnish with sriracha to taste.

Variation: Add 1 cup of cooked edamame just before serving.

Storage: Store in an airtight container for up to 5 days in the refrigerator.

NUTRITION INFORMATION
PER SERVING: Calories 250; Fat 9g (Sat 1g); Protein 7g; Carb 36g; Fiber 7g; Calcium 35mg; Iron 1.7mg; Sodium 140mg; Folate 28mcg
ALLERGENS: Wheat, Soy
* = Gluten Free Option

FERTILITY FOCUS: Whole grain noodles are an excellent way to enjoy your favorite foods while still promoting a fertility-fueling diet. Look for brands that list "100% whole grain" on the container, and focus on adding flavor with spices, healthy oils, and vegetables. Whole grains have not only been shown to increase your chances of fertility, but are also a great component of a healthy lifestyle.

Mexican Black Beans from Scratch

MAKES: 12 servings, ½ cup each
GLUTEN FREE, VEGAN

With just a little planning, delicious black beans can be yours, to be used in any meal. These beans freeze well, so enjoy some now or freeze them for a grab-and-go meal.

1 pound dried black beans, sorted
  and rinsed
1 tablespoon olive oil
1 yellow onion, chopped
1 tablespoon cumin seeds
6 cups water
3 cloves garlic, peeled and left whole
1 bay leaf
2 teaspoons kosher salt

Place rinsed beans in one or two large, sealable container(s). Pour water over beans, allowing a few inches of space for beans to expand and soak overnight in the refrigerator.

When ready to prepare the beans, heat the oil in a large pot set over medium heat. Add the onion and cook until softened, about 5 minutes. Add cumin seeds and cook an additional 1 minute, stirring constantly.

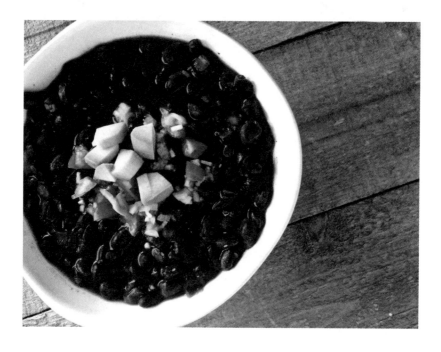

Drain the beans from the soaking liquid (discard liquid) and return to the pot with onions and cumin. Add the water, garlic, and bay leaf. Bring to a boil. Stir, then reduce the heat to a simmer and partially cover. Cook, stirring occasionally, for about 50 minutes to 1 hour. Add the salt and cook an additional 15 to 20 minutes, or until the beans are tender but still holding their shape.

Remove beans from heat and enjoy.

Variation: For a more authentic flavor, add 1 teaspoon Mexican oregano to the beans once you've removed them from the heat.

Storage: Refrigerate in an airtight container for up to 5 days. Freeze for up to 6 months.

NUTRITION INFORMATION
PER SERVING: Calories 150; Fat 2g (Sat 0g); Protein 8g; Carb 25g; Fiber 6g; Calcium 60mg; Iron 2.3mg; Sodium 330mg; Folate 170mcg

FERTILITY FOCUS: Plant proteins reign supreme in a fertility-fueling diet. Black beans are filled with protein and fiber, two things that will keep you satiated on this fertility roller coaster.

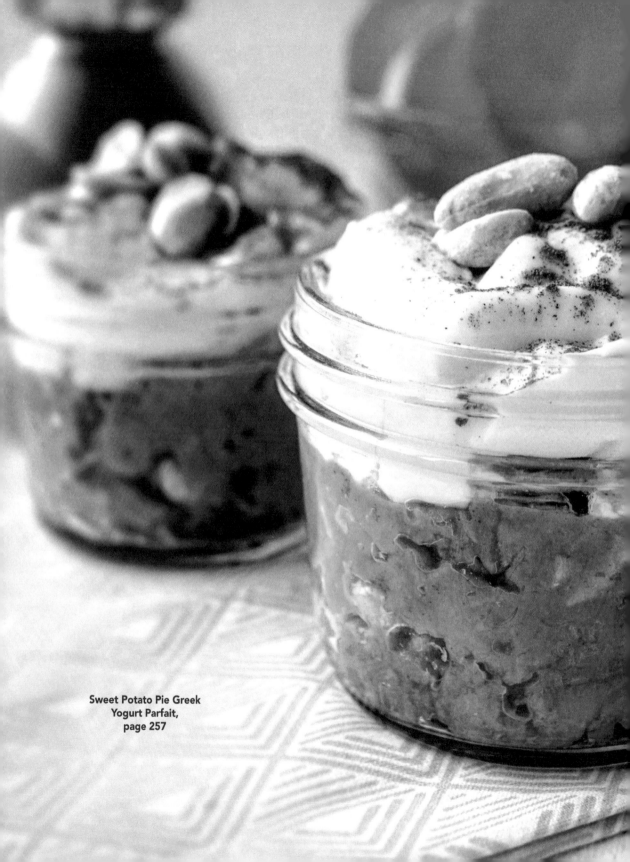

Sweet Potato Pie Greek
Yogurt Parfait,
page 257

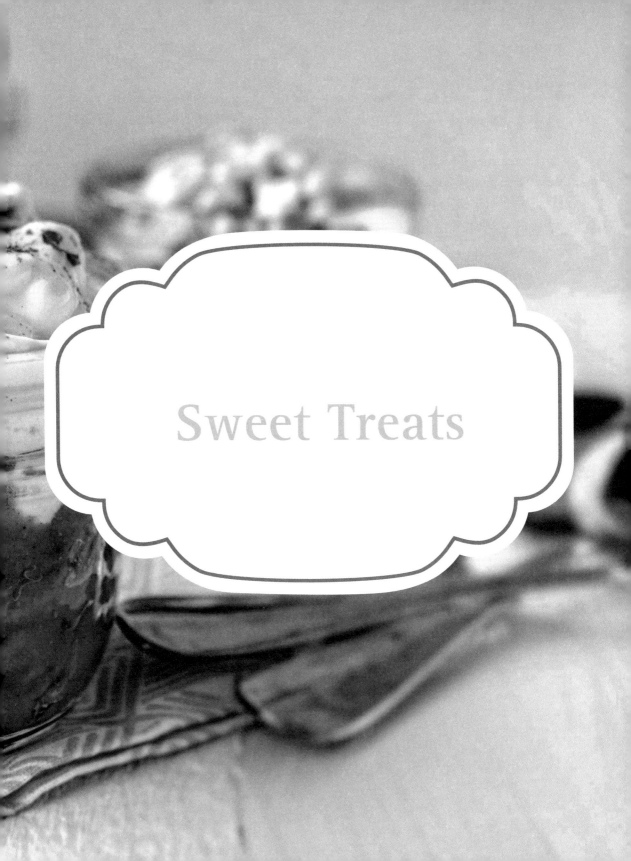

W E BOTH LOVE SWEET treats—and we've found ways to naturally satisfy our cravings *without* relying on highly processed foods filled with added sugars.

Though we encourage you to focus on fueling your bodies first with wholesome fruits and vegetables, we know sometimes that just doesn't cut it. That's why we've made these recipes—for those times when a little chocolate is just what you need!

Since that need for something sweet can come upon you fast, here are some quick ideas to throw together that satisfy that late night sweet tooth!

NATURALLY SWEET FOODS	SIMPLE SWEET TREAT
Banana	Slice banana in half, add 1 tablespoon Natural Peanut Butter (page 59) and top with a sprinkling of shaved dark chocolate.
Frozen Yogurt Grapes	Dip fresh grapes into a lightly sweetened yogurt and freeze.
Dates and Figs	A source of naturally-present sugar, these are nature's candy. We like to slice them in half and put a teaspoon of nut butter or goat cheese in between.

Banana Mango Sorbet with Toasted Coconut

F **MAKES: 4 servings of 1 cup each (4 cups)**
GLUTEN FREE, VEGAN

A light and refreshing frozen treat! With no added sugar, this sorbet is the perfect snack to wow your taste buds while delivering a hearty dose of vitamin C.

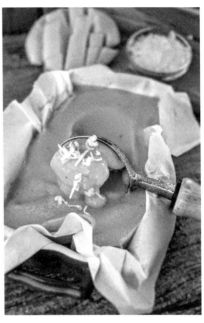

15 ounces (about 4 cups) frozen mango chunks
3 large (15 ounces) ripe bananas, peeled
4 tablespoons toasted and shredded sweetened coconut, divided

In a food processor or blender, puree frozen mangos until smooth, about 3 to 5 minutes. Add bananas and pulse another minute.

Transfer puree to sealed container and freeze for a minimum of 2 hours.

When ready to eat, remove from freezer 5 minutes prior to serving. Scoop into bowls and garnish with toasted coconut.

Variation: Use a scoop of sorbet in a smoothie (page 142) for a tropical kick!

Storage: Store in an airtight container in the freezer for up to 2 months.

NUTRITION INFORMATION
PER SERVING: Calories 170; Fat 2g (Sat 1.5g); Protein 2g; Carb 39g; Fiber 4g; Calcium 5mg; Iron 1.3mg; Sodium 15g; Folate 18mcg
ALLERGENS: Tree Nuts

FERTILITY FOCUS: Getting adequate vitamin C is important to make sure your body has a strong immune system. We don't need research to tell us this; it's ingrained in us from childhood, right? The cool thing about this combo is that it also delivers potassium, an essential nutrient crucial for blood pressure control and your overall health.

Tropical Chia Rice Pudding

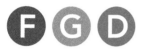

MAKES: 4 servings, ½ cup each
GLUTEN FREE, VEGETARIAN

Full of antioxidants, vitamins, and minerals, this sweet treat is almost too good to be true! For a fun twist, top pudding with the Zesty Mango Preserves (page 58).

1 cup water
½ cup brown rice, rinsed
¼ teaspoon kosher salt
⅔ cup whole milk
2 tablespoons + 1 teaspoon honey
½ teaspoon ground cinnamon
1 teaspoon vanilla extract
3 tablespoons chia seeds
1 cup chopped pineapple, divided
2 tablespoons chopped roasted,
    salted pistachios, divided

Pour water over brown rice in a medium pot. Add salt and cook over high heat until water begins to boil. Reduce heat to low, cover, and cook for about 30 minutes. Water should be fully absorbed and rice should be soft and chewy.

Drain any excess water and set rice in medium bowl. Add milk, honey, cinnamon, vanilla extract, and chia seeds to the bowl, stirring together until combined. Cover and set in the refrigerator for at least 2 hours to allow chia seeds to absorb milk and honey.

When ready to serve, portion pudding into bowls, then top with pineapple chunks and chopped pistachios.

Storage: Refrigerate for up to 2 days in a sealed container.

NUTRITION INFORMATION
PER SERVING: Calories 240; Fat 7g (Sat 1g); Protein 6g; Carb 40g; Fiber 6g; Calcium 116mg; Iron 1.4mg; Sodium 40mg; Folate 13mcg
ALLERGENS: Milk, Tree Nuts

FERTILITY FOCUS: Chia seeds are an excellent way to add omega-3 fatty acids into your diet, especially if you don't like seafood. Omega-3 fatty acids have been shown to help boost your mood, something we know we need every now and then on this journey!

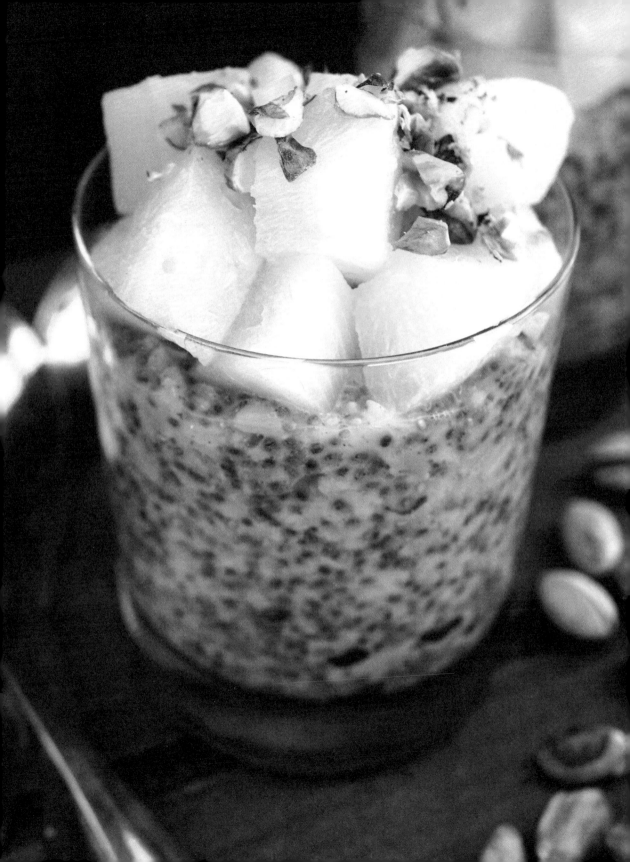

Dark Chocolate Cherry Almond "Bonbons"

(F) **MAKES: 5 servings, 3 portions each**
GLUTEN FREE, VEGAN

A simple dessert that will please any chocolate-loving palate!

15 ripe, sweet cherries, pitted
1 ounce 60 percent dark chocolate,
    broken into 15 pieces
2 tablespoons roasted and salted
    sliced almonds

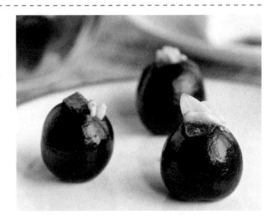

Place a small piece of dark chocolate in the pitted portion of each cherry.

Place cherries on a microwave safe plate and cover with a napkin. Microwave on high power for 10 seconds. If chocolate is not slightly melted, return to the microwave and cook an additional 5 seconds at a time until softened.

Remove from the microwave and add 3 to 4 sliced almonds to the pitted portion of each cherry. Serve immediately.

Variation: Use dark chocolate chips in place of chopped dark chocolate.

Kitchen Tip: Use a cherry pitter to remove cherry pits. No cherry pitter? No problem! Try using a chopstick or straw to push out the pit.

NUTRITION INFORMATION
PER SERVING: Calories 60; Fat 3.5g (Sat 1.5g); Protein 1g; Carb 7g; Fiber 1g; Calcium 13mg; Iron 0.5mg; Sodium 0mg; Folate 2mcg
ALLERGENS: Tree Nuts, Milk

FERTILITY FOCUS: Cherries contain anthocyanins, a type of flavonoid (or phyto-nutrient) that helps rid your body of harmful free radicals.

Cinnamon Raisin Oatmeal Cookies

MAKES: 30 cookies
GLUTEN FREE*, VEGETARIAN

A classic oatmeal cookie made with raisins and plenty of cinnamon. Enjoy these cookies with a cold glass of milk.

½ cup all-purpose flour^{GF}

½ cup white whole wheat flour^{GF}

½ teaspoon baking soda

¼ teaspoon baking powder

¾ teaspoon ground cinnamon

¼ teaspoon kosher salt

½ cup butter, softened

⅓ cup granulated sugar

⅓ cup packed brown sugar

1 large egg

1 teaspoon vanilla extract

½ cup (2 ounces) raisins (or alternative dried fruit)

¾ cup rolled old fashioned oats^{GF}

¼ cup (1 ounce) chopped pecans (optional)

Preheat the oven to 350°F and line 2 to 3 baking sheets with parchment paper.

In medium bowl, whisk together the flours, baking soda, baking powder, cinnamon, and salt. Set aside.

In a separate bowl, use a hand or stand mixer to whip the butter until creamy, about 2 to 3 minutes. Scrape down the sides of the bowl and add the granulated sugar and brown sugar. Blend about 1 to 2 minutes.

Add the egg and vanilla and mix until combined, about 20 seconds. Scrape down the sides of the bowl again, then add the dry ingredients. Blend on low speed until just combined. Add the dried fruit, oats, and nuts and mix until just combined.

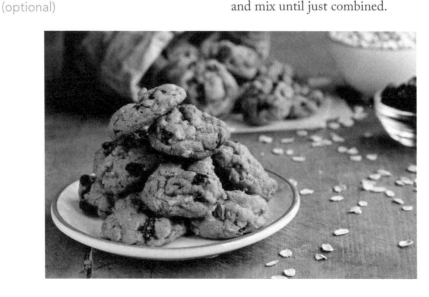

Drop dough by the rounded spoonful 2 inches apart on the prepared baking sheets. Bake for 10 to 12 minutes, or until golden. Allow to cool slightly on the pan before moving to a rack to cool.

Storage: Place in a sealed container in the pantry for up to 10 days. Freeze for up to 1 month.

NUTRITION INFORMATION
PER SERVING: Calories 80; Fat 4g (Sat 2g); Protein 1g; Carb 11g; Fiber 1g; Calcium 16mg; Iron 0.4mg; Sodium 95mg; Folate 6mcg
ALLERGENS: Wheat, Milk, Egg, Tree Nuts
* = Gluten Free Option

FERTILITY FOCUS: Limiting your intake of added sugars helps prevent blood sugar highs and lows, which is important for optimum fertility. Stocking your freezer with lower sugar, complex carbohydrate-based sweets to grab when a craving strikes is a great way to honor your sweet tooth while on your fertility journey.

Right Sized Chocolate Chip Cookie

MAKES: 20 cookies
GLUTEN FREE*, VEGETARIAN

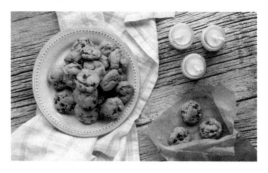

Everyone loves a fresh-baked chocolate chip cookie! These Right Sized Chocolate Chip Cookies are the perfect way to satisfy your sweet tooth while getting a dose of whole grains, too!

¾ cup all-purpose flour^{GF}
¾ cup white whole wheat flour^{GF}
½ teaspoon baking soda
¼ teaspoon kosher salt
1 stick salted butter, softened
⅓ cup packed brown sugar
⅓ cup granulated sugar
1 large egg
1 teaspoon pure vanilla extract
½ cup (4 ounces) mini chocolate chips

NUTRITION INFORMATION
PER SERVING: Calories 130; Fat 7g (Sat 4g); Protein 2g; Carb 18g; Fiber 1g; Calcium 26mg; Iron 0.7mg; Sodium 160mg; Folate 11mcg
ALLERGENS: Wheat, Milk, Egg
* = Gluten Free Option

Preheat the oven to 350°F and line two large baking sheets with parchment paper.

In a medium bowl, combine the flours, baking soda, and salt.

In a large bowl, add the softened butter. Using a hand or stand mixer, mix for about 1 minute on medium speed. Scrape down the sides of the bowl and add the sugars. Mix for another 2 minutes on high speed, until the mixture is light and fluffy. Add the egg and vanilla extract and mix until just combined, about 30 seconds or so. Scrape down the bowl.

Reduce the mixer speed to low and add the flour mixture, mixing until combined. Scrape down the bowl and stir in the chocolate chips.

Roll ½-ounce portions of cookie dough balls (about a tablespoon) and place on the baking sheets. Bake until lightly browned, about 8 to 11 minutes. Remove from the pans and cool on a rack.

Storage: Place in a sealed container in the pantry for up to 10 days. Freeze for up to 1 month.

FERTILITY FOCUS: Managing stress helps you achieve your most fertile self. Eliminating foods you like, such as cookies, will not solve your infertility. Instead, focus on including better for you treats (i.e., lower in added sugar) when you want something sweet in the proper portion.

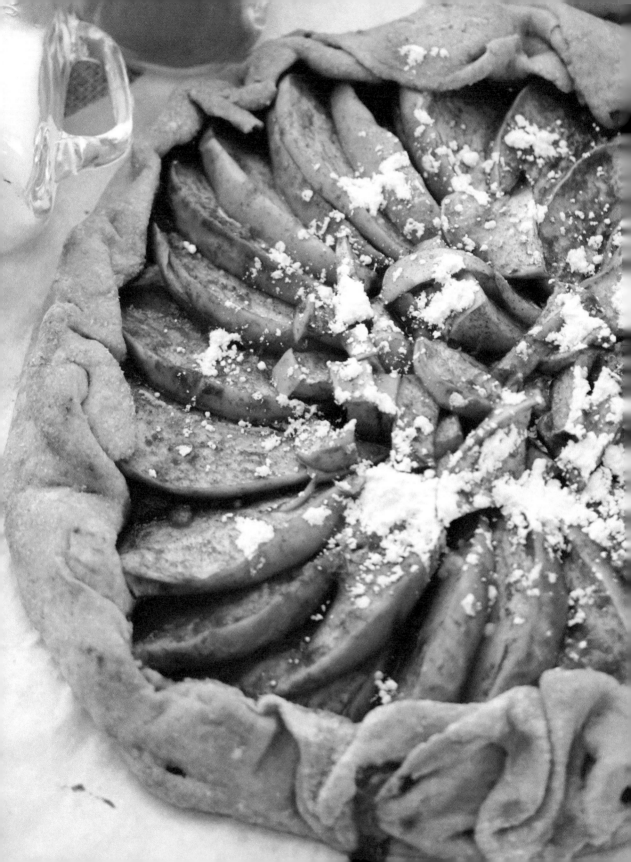

Rustic Apple Galette

MAKES: 8-inch galette, 8 servings, 1 slice each
GLUTEN FREE*, VEGETARIAN

A galette. Sounds fancy, right? Don't worry; it's actually very simple to make! A galette is a flat round dough filled with fruit (in sweet versions) or potatoes and vegetables (in savory options). This rustic apple galette is low in sugar and incorporates whole grain flour and plenty of delicious, fiber filling apples.

Dough (makes about 7½ ounces dough)

¼ cup lightly scooped all-purpose flour^{GF}

⅓ cup lightly scooped white whole wheat flour^{GF}

¼ teaspoon kosher salt

1 tablespoon granulated sugar

6 tablespoons cold salted butter, cut into small cubes

1 to 2 tablespoons cold water

Filling

2 tablespoons packed brown sugar

1 teaspoon ground cinnamon

⅛ teaspoon ground nutmeg

1 tablespoon cornstarch

1 tablespoon lemon juice

1 teaspoon granulated sugar

1 pound granny smith or apple of choice (about 3 medium apples)

1 teaspoon diced salted butter

To make the dough, combine the flours, salt and sugar in a food processor and pulse 5 times. Toss in the cold butter and pulse an additional 15 to 20 times, until butter is combined and mixture resembles coarse sand. Add the water, all at once with the processor's motor running, then stop and pulse 2 to 3 times, or until dough just comes together. Shape dough into a disc, wrap in plastic wrap and refrigerate until cold, about 1 hour.

Preheat the oven to 400°F. Line a baking sheet with parchment paper. Remove the dough from the fridge and, on a well-floured surface, roll the dough out into a 10-inch circle. Brush off excess flour and transfer dough to the prepared baking sheet.

In a large bowl, combine the brown sugar, cinnamon and nutmeg. Remove 1 tablespoon of the mixture and set aside. Add cornstarch and lemon juice to the large bowl and then peel, core and slice the apples into ¼-inch slices and add them to the bowl. Toss to combine.

Place the apple mixture in the middle of the dough, leaving a 1½-inch border. Sprinkle the reserved cinnamon sugar mixture over the apples and dot with remaining diced butter. Carefully fold the dough over the apples, pleating the dough to make a circle. Tent a piece of foil loosely over the galette and bake for 20 minutes. Remove the foil and bake an additional 20 minutes.

Variation: Refrigerated pie dough can be substituted for the homemade dough, but note that nutrition values will change.

Storage: The dough can be made a day in advance. Refrigerate for up to 3 days.

Kitchen Tip: Brush the edges of the dough with egg wash before baking to give the crust a golden sheen. To make the egg wash, mix 1 large egg with 1 tablespoon water and brush a thin coat lightly onto dough.

NUTRITION INFORMATION
PER SERVING: Calories 150; Fat 9g (Sat 6g); Protein 1g; Carb 18g; Fiber 2g; Calcium 17mg; Iron 0.3mg; Sodium 140mg; Folate 6mcg
ALLERGENS: Wheat, Milk
* = Gluten Free Option

FERTILITY FOCUS: The beauty of the galette is that it has less "crust" as compared to a typical two crust pie. That means there's more room for apples! This dessert just makes sense and is a great alternative to other sugar-laden pies and sweet treats.

Sweet Potato Pie Greek Yogurt Parfait

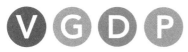

MAKES: 2 parfaits
GLUTEN FREE, VEGETARIAN

This Sweet Potato Pie Yogurt Parfait has that sweet goodness you crave with minimal added sugar. You can easily serve this as an afternoon snack or, if you're looking for a late night sweet treat, this makes a great dessert with Maple Cinnamon Walnuts (page 133).

1 medium sweet potato (or 1 cup sweet potato puree)
¼ teaspoon cinnamon
¼ teaspoon vanilla extract
2 tablespoons chopped pecans, divided (or nut of choice)
1 cup plain whole milk Greek yogurt (divided into ½ cups)
1 teaspoon maple syrup (optional)

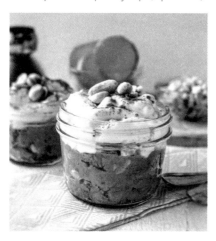

Preheat oven to 375°F. Poke sweet potato all over with a fork, wrap in foil and bake for 30 to 40 minutes, or until soft. Let cool. (skip this step if using sweet potato puree)

Remove sweet potato skin and beat sweet potato using electric mixer until smooth. Add cinnamon and vanilla extract. Stir in 1 tablespoon of chopped pecans. Divide sweet potato puree into half portions and place in bottom of small jars and cover with ½ cup Greek yogurt. Top with remaining pecans and a drizzle of maple syrup, if desired. Serve immediately.

Kitchen Tip: Microwaving your potatoes for 4 to 5 minutes prior to baking can speed up the cooking process. Puncture potato with a fork prior to microwaving.

NUTRITION INFORMATION
PER SERVING: Calories 250; Fat 10g (Sat 3.5g); Protein 13g; Carb 29g; Fiber 4g; Calcium 175mg; Iron 0.9mg; Sodium 280mg; Folate 8mcg
ALLERGENS: Milk, Tree Nuts, Peanuts

FERTILITY FOCUS: Sweet potatoes are filled with vitamin A, an important fat-soluble vitamin that needs to be consumed with a dietary fat to get the most "bang for your buck," nutritionally speaking. By combining whole milk Greek yogurt and heart healthy monounsaturated nuts in this parfait, you get the best of both worlds (sweet and salty) to fuel your fertility!

Berrylicious Fruit Crumble

MAKES: 8 servings, ½ cup each
GLUTEN FREE*, VEGETARIAN

Fruit crumbles are also a great way to add an extra serving of fruit to your day. The natural sugars of fruit caramelize beautifully when baked.

Fruit Filling
2½ cups strawberries, chopped
  (fresh or frozen, about 16 ounces)
1 cup raspberries (fresh or frozen,
  6 ounces)
1 tablespoon granulated sugar
1½ teaspoons lemon juice
½ teaspoon lemon zest
2 tablespoons white whole wheat
  flour^{GF}

Oat Crumble Topping
2 tablespoons white whole wheat
  flour^{GF}
⅔ cup rolled old fashioned oats^{GF}
1 tablespoon brown sugar, packed
¾ teaspoon ground cinnamon
¼ teaspoon kosher salt
1 tablespoon melted butter
  (or 1 tablespoon vegetable oil)
1 tablespoon whole milk
1½ teaspoon vanilla extract
2 tablespoons chopped walnuts

Preheat oven to 375°F. In a medium bowl, mix together strawberries, raspberries, sugar, lemon juice and lemon zest. Place fruit mixture into a 9-inch pie pan sprayed with nonstick spray. Cover with foil and bake for 20 minutes.

While baking, mix flour, oats, brown sugar, cinnamon and salt in a bowl, and set aside. In a small bowl, whisk together the butter (or vegetable oil), milk and vanilla. Pour the wet ingredients into the dry and blend together using the back of a fork as a pastry blender, mixing until dry ingredients are well coated.

Mix in the chopped walnuts and sprinkle the remaining oat crumble topping over the top of the pie dish. Continue to bake, uncovered, for remaining 15 to 20 minutes, until fruit bubbles at the top. Remove and let cool for 10 to 15 minutes before serving.

Variation: Substitute 1½ pounds pitted sweet cherries, cut in half, ½ teaspoon almond extract for vanilla extract, and sliced almonds for the walnuts.

Storage: Refrigerate in a sealed container for up to 3 days.

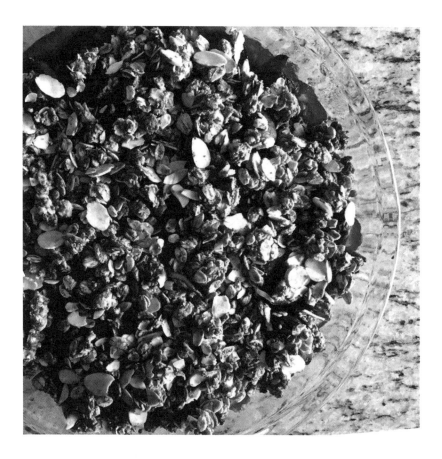

NUTRITION INFORMATION

PER SERVING: Calories 110; Fat 3.5g (Sat 0g); Protein 2g; Carb 17g; Fiber 3g; Calcium 21mg; Iron 0.8mg; Sodium 60mg; Folate 17mcg

ALLERGENS: Wheat, Milk, Tree Nuts

* = Gluten Free Option

FERTILITY FOCUS: This dessert is low in added sugar and is topped with whole grain oats, which makes it better than many of its crumble competitors. Research shows high intakes of the antioxidants found in fruit, like berries, are a great addition to a fertility fueling diet.

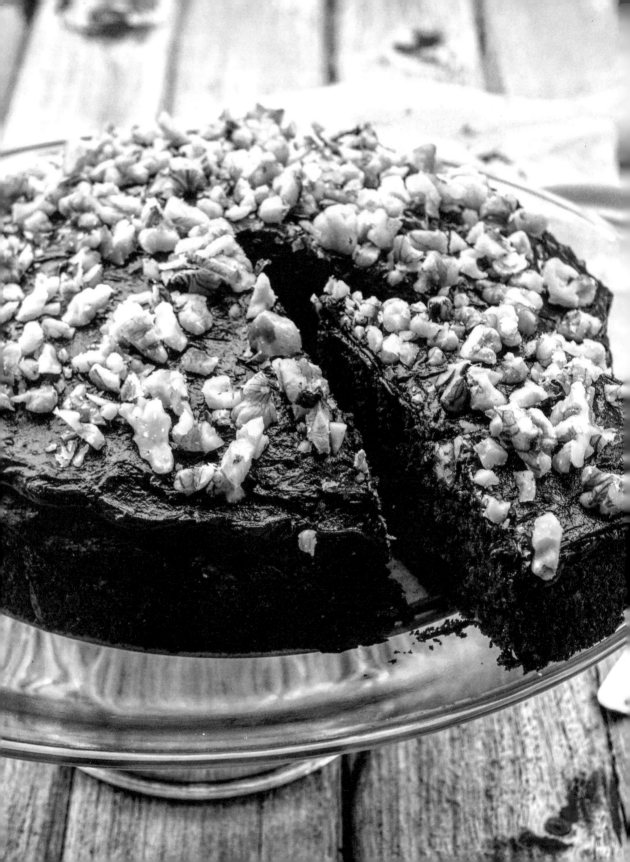

Heavenly Chocolate Cake with Rich and Creamy Chocolate Frosting

MAKES: 9-inch cake, 8 servings, 1 slice each
GLUTEN FREE*,
VEGETARIAN

You can make a decadent chocolate cake using just a few ingredients, one which may even be in your garden! We snuck in an extra dose of fiber and vitamins by adding grated zucchini, which creates a rich, moist cake. Rest easy knowing you're filling your body with a lower sugar cake, filled with flavor and that chocolatey goodness you crave.

Chocolate Cake

1½ cups (1 medium zucchini, 5 ounces approximately) zucchini
⅔ cup whole milk
1 teaspoon apple cider vinegar
1⅔ cups white whole wheat flour, sifted^{GF}
⅔ cup cocoa powder (dark for a richer flavor)
1½ teaspoons baking soda
½ teaspoon baking powder
¼ teaspoon kosher salt
⅔ cup granulated sugar
⅓ cup vegetable oil
2 teaspoons vanilla extract
2 large eggs

Frosting

⅖ medium (2 ounces) avocado
¼ cup powdered sugar
2 ½ tablespoons cocoa powder (dark for a richer flavor)
2 tablespoons whole milk
1 ounce Roasted Mixed Nuts (page 130) (or alternative nut), chopped

Preheat oven to 350°F. Coat an 8-inch spring form pan with cooking spray.

Peel and shred the zucchini into a small bowl. Set aside.

In a measuring cup, combine milk and apple cider vinegar, set aside for 10 minutes. In a medium bowl, combine flour, cocoa powder, baking soda, baking powder and salt. Set aside.

In a large bowl, add the sugar, oil, vanilla and eggs. Whisk together until thoroughly combined. Add milk and vinegar mixture to the bowl with the sugar and stir. Gently fold in the zucchini. Add the flour mixture, stirring until combined.

Pour the batter into the prepared pan. Place in the oven and bake for 30 to 35 minutes, or until a toothpick comes out clean from the center. Remove from oven and let the pan cool on a wire rack.

In a small bowl, using a hand mixer on medium speed, blend avocado until smooth. On low speed, mix in the powdered sugar, cocoa powder and milk. Continue to mix until smooth and incorporated. Set aside.

Once cake has cooled, frost cake and garnish with chopped nuts.

Variation: Use an 8 x 8-inch square pan lined with parchment paper. Bake for 25 to 30 minutes, or until wooden pick comes out clean when inserted in the center.

Storage: Place in an airtight container in the refrigerator for up to 2 days. Freeze for up to 4 months.

Kitchen Tip: Avocados are a great alternative to butter in baking. They have the creamy, smooth consistency of butter but are filled with heart healthy fats!

NUTRITION INFORMATION
PER SERVING: Calories 370; Fat 16g (Sat 3g); Protein 8g; Carb 48mg; Fiber 7g; Calcium 87mg; Iron 2.6mg; Sodium 390mg; Folate 23mcg
ALLERGENS: Milk, Wheat, Egg, Tree Nuts, Peanuts
* = Gluten Free Option

FERTILITY FOCUS: This cake packs a whopping 7 grams of protein and is made with 100 percent whole grains, meaning your blood sugars won't skyrocket post-indulgence like a traditional chocolate cake. Keeping your body in balance, especially your blood sugars, is crucial for your fertility.

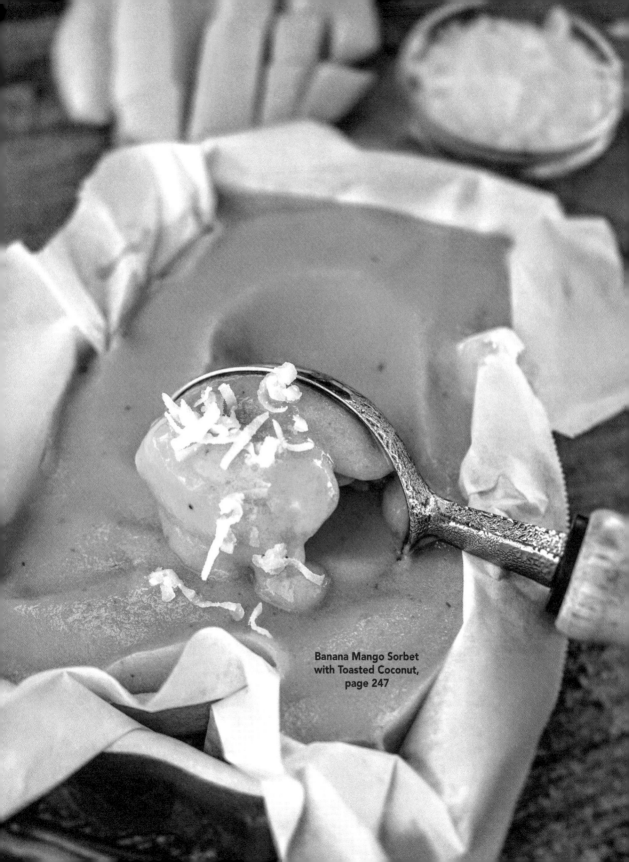

Banana Mango Sorbet
with Toasted Coconut,
page 247

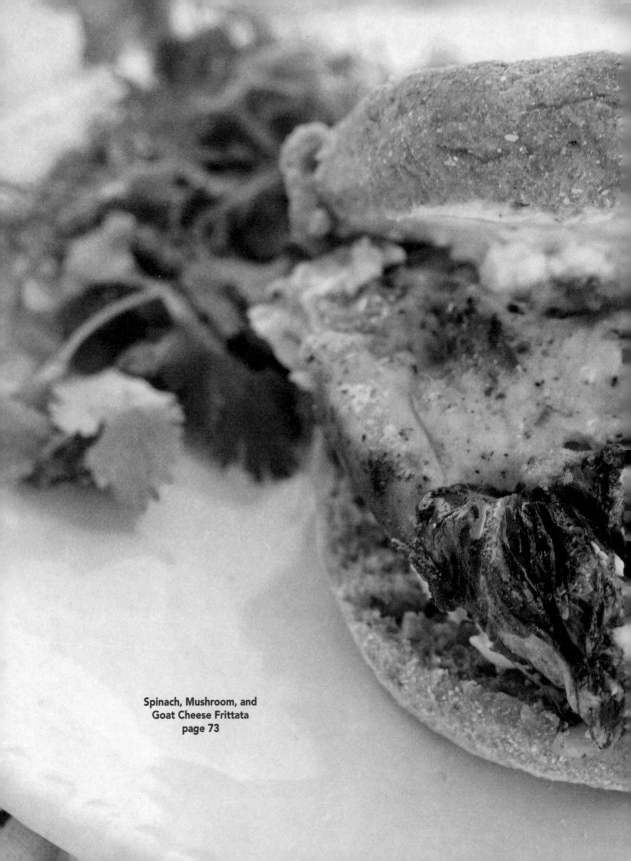

Spinach, Mushroom, and
Goat Cheese Frittata
page 73

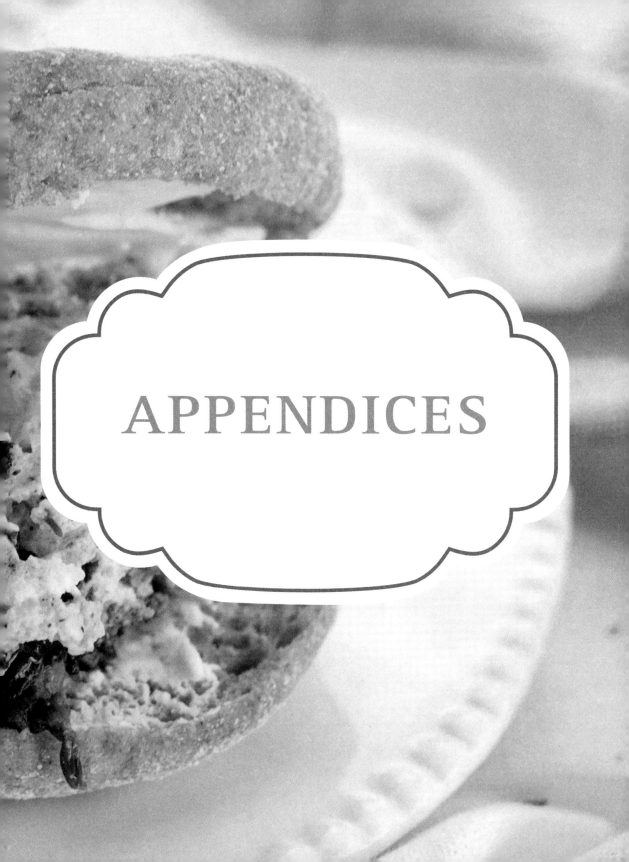

APPENDICES

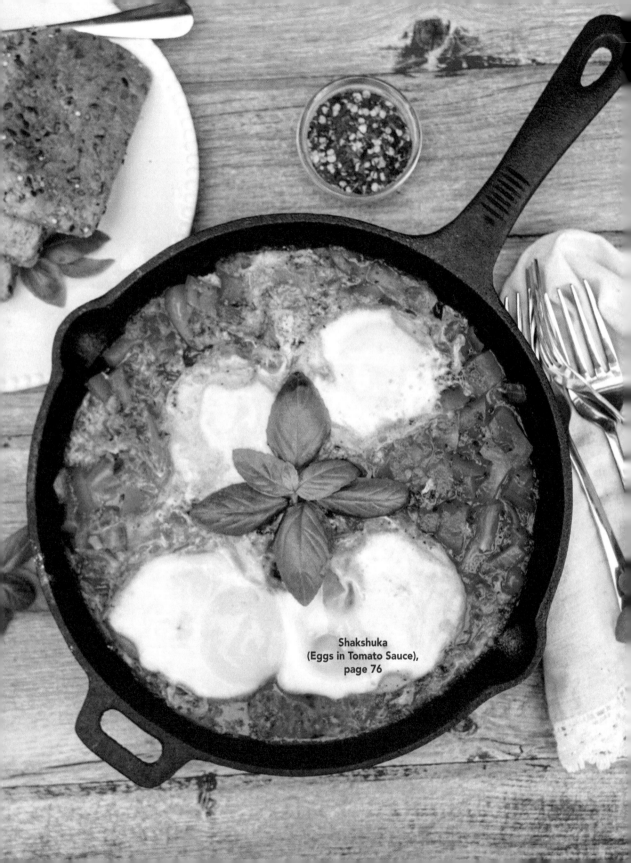

Shakshuka
(Eggs in Tomato Sauce),
page 76

APPENDIX A:
DIETARY REFERENCE INTAKE FOR
ADULT MALES AND FEMALES (AGES 19 TO 50)[38]

Dietary Reference Intakes (DRIs) refers to the amount of nutrients (including vitamins and minerals) that individuals are recommended to consume on a daily basis (RDA and AI referenced).

NUTRIENT	Females Ages 19 to 30 years	Females Ages 31 to 50 years	Males Ages 19 to 30 years	Males Ages 31 to 50 years
Protein (g)	46	46	56	56
Carbohydrates (g)	130	130	130	130
Fiber (g)	25	25	38	38
Vitamin A (mg)	700	700	900	900
Vitamin D (IU)	600	600	600	600
Vitamin E (mg)	15	15	15	15
Vitamin K (mg)	120	120	90	90
Vitamin C (mg)	75	75	90	90
Thiamin (mg)	1.1	1.1	1.2	1.2
Riboflavin (mg)	1.1	1.1	1.3	1.3
Niacin (mg)	14	14	16	16
Vitamin B6 (mg)	1.3	1.3	1.3	1.3
Folate (mcg)	400	400	400	400
Vitamin B12 (mg)	2.4	2.4	2.4	2.4
Iron (mg)	18	18	8	8
Calcium (mg)	1000	1000	1000	1000
Phosphorus (mg)	700	700	700	700
Magnesium (mg)	310	320	400	420
Zinc (mg)	8	8	11	11
Iodine (mg)	150	150	150	150
Biotin (mg)	30	30	30	30
Choline (mg)	425	425	550	550
Selenium (mg)	55	55	55	55
Sodium (mg)	1500	1500	1500	1500
Potassium (mg)	4700	4700	4700	4700
α-linolenic acid (g)	1.1*	1.1*	1.6*	1.6*
Linoleic acid (g)	12*	12*	17*	17*

* = Adequate Intake (AI)

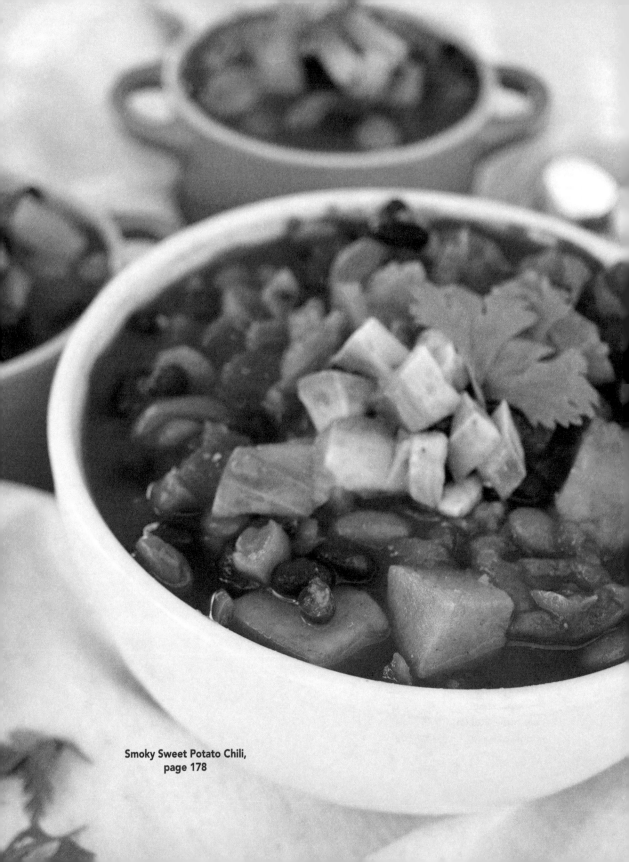

Smoky Sweet Potato Chili,
page 178

APPENDIX B:
BUILDING A HEALTHY KITCHEN: THE STAPLES

TIPS FOR SUCCESS

- Make a list before you shop!
- Use this list as a guide to fill your pantry, refrigerator and freezer.
- Embrace trying new foods, flavors and recipes!

PRODUCE

Pre-washed, bagged spinach, kale, mixed greens

Romaine hearts

Bananas

Apples

Berries (whatever is in season)

Summer squash, including yellow squash and zucchini

Avocados

Mushrooms

Onions (yellow, white or red)

Sweet potatoes

Tomatoes

Carrots

Fresh herbs (dill, cilantro, rosemary, thyme, oregano, basil)

FROZEN PRODUCE

Frozen mixed vegetables (broccoli, cauliflower, carrot blend and stir fry blend)

Frozen berries (without added sugar)

Shop the sales! Stock up on items you can make multiple meals out of.

GRAINS/BREADS

Navigating the grocery store in search of whole grain foods can sometimes feel like trying to find a needle in a haystack. Luckily for you, there are a few clues that let you know a product is a whole grain or contains whole grains. The chart below is a great reference you can use to evaluate if that item you're holding is a worthy "whole grain" choice.

> ### DOES THE PRODUCT...
>
> ✓ List 100 percent whole grains as the first ingredient?
>
> ✓ Have > 3 grams of fiber per serving ?
>
> ✓ Contain the Whole Grain Stamp of Approval? [39]

100% whole wheat or whole grain bread	Whole grain oats/white whole wheat flour
100% whole wheat English muffin	High fiber/whole grain cereal
Corn tortillas (4-inch)	Amaranth/quinoa
Whole wheat flour tortillas (8-inch)	Wild rice/brown rice/couscous
Whole grain pitas (6-inch)	Whole wheat pasta

SNACK FOODS

Whole wheat/grain crackers	Unsalted, raw nuts (pistachios, almonds, walnuts, pine nuts)
Air popped popcorn	

DAIRY

Whole milk (or milk alternative if allergic to cow's milk)	Whole milk ricotta cheese
Plain, whole milk Greek yogurt	Shaved Parmesan cheese
Neufchatel cream cheese	Whole milk mozzarella cheese
4 percent fat large cottage cheese	Large eggs
	Margarine or butter (your choice)

ANIMAL PROTEINS

Boneless, skinless chicken breasts

Lean ground turkey

Mahi mahi/salmon filets

Frozen shrimp

Canned albacore tuna/salmon in water

ALTERNATIVE PROTEINS

Extra firm tofu

Beans, legumes, lentils

Quinoa, amaranth (see whole grains
    above)

All natural nut butters

Eggs/dairy (see above)

CONDIMENTS/PANTRY STAPLES

Ketchup, mustard

Low sodium soy sauce

Vegetable broth: low sodium

Canned tomatoes: no salt added

Spices (garlic, onion, parsley, basil,
    oregano, pepper, salt, cumin,
    paprika, cinnamon)

Taco sauce, hot sauce

Lemon or lime juice

Rice, balsamic and apple cider vinegar

Fast acting yeast

Baking powder, baking soda

Pure vanilla extract

Brown/white (or granulated) sugar

Unsweetened applesauce

Cooking spray

Olive oil

Canola oil (or vegetable oil of choice)

Pure maple syrup

Honey

COOKING GADGETS

Wooden spoons	Mixing bowls
Spatula	Microplane
Measuring cups and spoons	Box grater
Chef's knife	Sauce pots
Paring knife	Sauté pans
Blender or immersion blender	Dutch oven or large pot
Whisk	Cast iron pan
Cutting boards	Tongs
Sheet pans	Colander

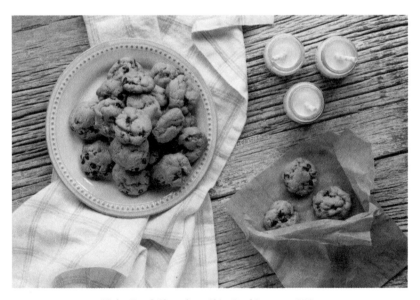

Right Sized Chocolate Chip Cookie, page 253

APPENDIX C:
COOKING TECHNIQUES AND TERMS

Technique	Definition	Good For
Bake	Dry-heat method*; food is cooked with hot, dry air; food is cooked at a lower temperature than what is used for roasting	Vegetables, fruits, poultry, and fish
Boil	Moist-heat method**; food is cooked in a hot liquid such as water or broth	Cooking pasta and whole grains
Broil	Dry-heat method; food is cooked using heat from an above source	Fruits, vegetables, and tender cuts of meat
Brown	Cooking with fat over high heat with the intention of adding color or caramelization to the food	Vegetables, poultry, and meat
Grill	Dry-heat cooking method where heat source is below	Fruits, vegetables, and tender cuts of meat
Roast	Dry-heat method; food is cooked with hot, dry air; typically heat is higher than baking, resulting in more browning	Vegetables and larger cuts of meat
Sauté	Dry-heat method; relies on fat (typically oil or butter) to quickly cook food over medium to high heat	Vegetables and tender cuts of meat
Steam	Moist-heat method; gently cooks food using steam, whereby water does not directly touch the food; requires no fat	Fruits, vegetables, fish, and poultry
Sweat	Cooking with a small amount of fat, usually over lower heat with the intention of softening the food without browning	Typically used for vegetable cookery

* Dry-heat method refers to the cooking technique where heat is directly transferred to the food, without the presence of moisture.
** Moist-heat method refers to the cooking technique where liquid is used to cook the food.

ESSENTIAL KNIFE CUTS

KNIFE CUT	SIZE/SHAPE	IMAGE
Chop (rough)	Food is cut into roughly the same size, bite-shaped pieces.	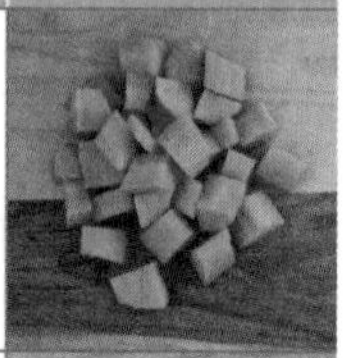
Chop (fine) or mince	Food is cut into roughly the same size pieces, which are much smaller/finer than a rough chop	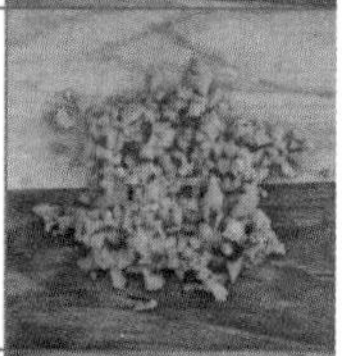
Dice, large	Food is cut into ¾ inch x ¾ inch x ¾ inch	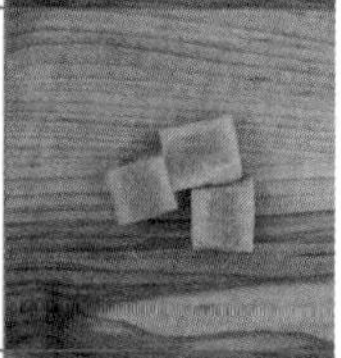
Dice, medium	½ inch x ½ inch x ½ inch	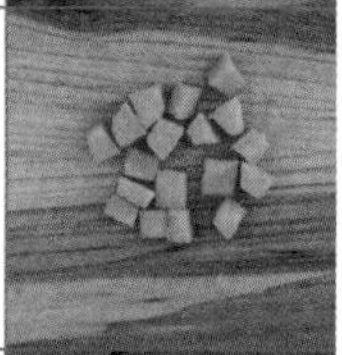
Dice, small	¼ inch x ¼ inch x ¼ inch	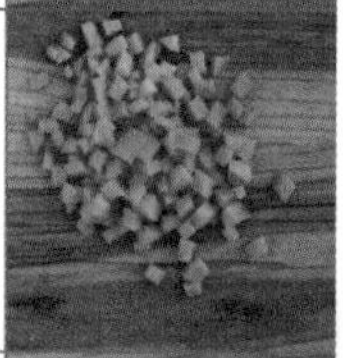
Julienne	Food is cut into thin strips, ⅛ inch x ⅛ inch x ⅛ inch	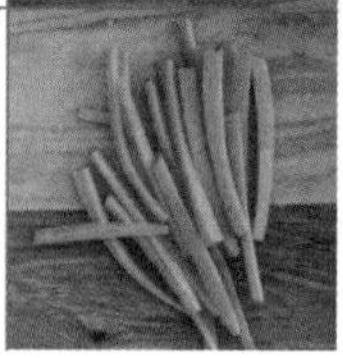

APPENDIX D:
FOOD SAFETY RECOMMENDATIONS[36,37]

Are you practicing proper food safety? When struggling with fertility, the last thing your body needs is to be exposed to a foodborne illness! Let's keep those foreign invaders out of our systems by practicing these simple steps. Remember, food safety involves *all* aspects of food preparation, from the moment you buy the food to the second you reheat those leftovers.

AT THE MARKET

Shop for your dry foods first, and then end your trip by picking up refrigerated and frozen foods. Bring insulated bags and ice packs to safely transport these foods home. Wrap your raw meats, including seafood, in bags so they don't drip onto your other items during transport. Consider designating one bag specifically for these items.

STORING FOOD

Have you ever heard of the term FIFO? If not, here's a quick education for you! FIFO stands for "first in, first out," meaning whatever you opened or bought first (or is expiring first) should be what you use/cook with first. This is important if you're one of those people who likes to "stock up" on certain items. Labeling and dating your foods can help with this.

Remember to keep the raw meats, poultry, and seafood on the very bottom of your refrigerator. You don't want the juice from your raw meat and seafood dripping onto your fresh produce, do you?

Here's a look at the proper way to stock your refrigerator, from the top down.

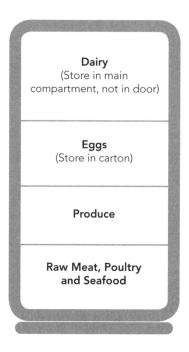

Dairy
(Store in main compartment, not in door)

Eggs
(Store in carton)

Produce

Raw Meat, Poultry and Seafood

Also, because we know you're not the only one out there confused about this, here's a quick reference for what those dates mean on your foods, and if they are still good to eat past those dates!

Term	Meaning	Past that date? Keep or Toss!
USE BY	The final date to consume for best quality. Designated by manufacturer of the product.	Toss! You're trying to make another person, right? Consume the best nourishment possible!
SELL BY	Date the store must sell the product by; can be consumed after purchase.	Keep, but be wise! Use within 2 to 3 days or toss.
BEST BY	Product is at its optimal quality until this date.	Toss! No comment needed!

For more information on this, please refer to the resources section (page 279) for information from the USDA.

What about leftovers? Cover and store leftover food within two hours of cooking, and toss if sitting out longer than that period. Foodborne bacteria can develop quickly when food is exposed to the temperature danger zone (41 to 135°F).

COOKING

Defrost. Safely defrost foods in the refrigerator or microwave, following package directions. Do not set foods on the counter to defrost, as this creates the perfect environment for bacteria to develop.

Wash, Clean, and Rinse. Wash and clean your hands with warm, soapy water first! Then, make sure your preparation area is clean. Rinse produce under water to remove dirt and debris. As for raw meats, poultry or seafood, there's no need to rinse, as this can actually spread bacteria, contaminating your sink and work surfaces.

Preparing. Take out your ingredients in the order you're going to need them. For instance, if you're preparing the Chicken Salad (page 122) but need to precook your chicken, do not take out your Greek yogurt until the chicken has been cooked and cooled. Leaving foods out of their recommended temperature zones for greater than two hours poses a serious risk of foodborne illness.

TEMPERATURES

Use this as a general guide to know what internal temperature the foods in this cookbook should reach when cooking!

Food	Internal Temperature
Poultry (chicken, turkey)	165°F
Fish (salmon, whitefish)	145°F
Shrimp	Cook until flesh is pearly and opaque
Reheating Leftovers	165°F

Other important tips:

- Store foods below 40°F in the refrigerator. This helps prevent the growth of bacteria.
- Purchase a kitchen thermometer! This is crucial to help ensure proper cooking temperatures are reached. (See Appendix for other useful cooking gadgets.)
- Purchase a refrigerator thermometer! This helps ensure the temperature inside is safely resting at 40°F or below.
- Wash your reusable totes often, and never set them on your kitchen countertops.
- Purchase separate cutting boards to prevent cross-contamination: one for produce, one for meat, one for poultry, and one for seafood. Discard boards when cracks or deep scratches appear, as these are potential areas for bacteria to breed.
- If all else fails, remember the age old adage still reigns true: *"When in doubt, throw it out!"*

(Reference: Food and Drug Administration, Academy Nutrition and Dietetics)

RESOURCES

ONLINE RESOURCES

USDA Food Safety
fsis.usda.gov

MyPlate.gov
www.choosemyplate.gov

Academy of Nutrition and Dietetics
www.eatright.org

Sara Haas RDN
http://www.sarahaasrdn.com

Shaw's Simple Swaps
http://shawsimpleswaps.com

Resolve: The National Infertility Association
http://www.resolve.org

Shine Fertility: A Support Group for Infertility
http://www.shinefertility.org

Bumps to Baby: A Community for Women with Infertility
http://www.bumpstobaby.com

NEDA (National Eating Disorder Awareness)
http://nedawareness.org

American Addiction Centers
http://americanaddictioncenters.org

Get Fit Now
http://www.getfitnow.com

BOOKS

Balch JF, Stengler M, Balch RY. *Prescription for Natural Cures: A self-care guide for treating health problems with natural remedies including diet, nutrition, supplements, and other holistic methods*. Revised ed. Hoboken, NJ: John Wiley and Sons, Inc., 2011.

Domar, A. *Conquering Infertility.* New York, NY: Penguin Books, 2004.

Rinaldi N, Buckler S, Waddell E and L. *No Period, Now What? A Guide to Regaining Your Cycles and Improving Your Fertility*. Waltham, MA: Antica Press LLC, 2016.

Ruder, Sonali. *Natural Pregnancy Cookbook*. New York: Hatherleigh Press, 2015.

Ruder, Sonali. *Natural Baby Food*. New York: Hatherleigh Press, 2016.

RESEARCH STUDIES

One of the benchmark studies referenced throughout the literature on fertility is the Nurses' Health Study II. This long-term research project followed more than 116,000 women between the ages of 25 and 42 to evaluate their lifestyle patterns and the corresponding risk of chronic disease. Dr. Walter Willett, a researcher from the Harvard School of Public Health, used this study to explore the reproductive health of women. Eighteen thousand females were selected out of the original sample based on their desire to conceive. The findings from this were then analyzed and interpreted by researchers from the Harvard School of Public Health and discussed in *The Fertility Diet*. Dr. Chavarro and team set forth the principles of a sound nutritional plan that included a predominately plant based diet, high in fiber, whole grains, whole milk dairy and healthy fats.

REFERENCES

1. Center for Disease Control Website. CDC. http://www.cdc.gov/reproductivehealth/infertility/. Updated September 16, 2015. Accessed March 6, 2016.

2. Campbell C, Jacobson H. *Whole: Rethinking the science of nutrition.* Dallas, TX: BenBella Books, Inc., 2013.

3. United States Department of Agriculture Website. Past Food Pyramid Materials. https://fnic.nal.usda.gov/dietary-guidance/myplate-and-historical-food-pyramid-resources/past-food-pyramid-materials. Updated March 4, 2016. Accessed February 26, 2016

4. United States Department of Agriculture Website. My Plate. http://www.choosemyplate.gov. Updated March 3, 2016. Accessed February 26, 2016.

5. Gaskins AJ, Colaci DS, Mendiola J, Swan SH, Chavarro JE. Dietary patterns and semen quality in young men. *Hum Reprod.* 2012; 27(10):2899-907. doi:10.1093/humrep/des298

6. Chiu YH, Afeiche MC, Gaskins AJ, et al. Fruit and vegetable intake and their pesticide residues in relation to semen quality among men from a fertility clinic. *Hum Reprod.* 2015;30(6):1342–1351. doi:10.1093/humrep/dev064.

7. Environmental Working Group Website. EWG's Summary. http://www.foodnews.org. Accessed July 18, 2016.

8. Winter CK, Katz JM. Dietary exposure to pesticide residues from commodities alleged to contain the highest contamination levels. *J Toxicol.* 2011. doi:10.1155 percent2F2011 percent2F589674.

9. Homan GF, Davies M, Norman R. The impact of lifestyle factors on reproductive performance in the general population and those undergoing infertility treatment: a review. *Human Reprod.* 2007;13(3):209-223. doi:10.1093/humupd/dml056.

10. Fruits and Veggies More Matters Website. http://www.fruitsandveggiesmorematters.org/what-are-phytochemicals. Updated February 10, 2012. Accessed July 29, 2016.

11. Rink SM, Mendola P, Mumford SL, et al. Self-Report of fruit and vegetable intake that meets the 5 a day recommendation is associated with reduced levels of oxidative stress biomarkers and increased levels of antioxidant defense in premenopausal women. *J Acad Nutr Diet.* 2013;113(6):776–785.

12. Today's Dietitian Website. Color Me Healthy. http://www.todaysdietitian.com/newarchives/110308p34.shtml. Updated November 2008. Accessed July 29, 2016.

13. Health Communications Core. Nurses Health Study. http://www.nurseshealthstudy.org/. Updated 2016. Accessed July-November 2016.

14. Chavarro JE, Willett WC, Skerrett PJ. *The Fertility Diet: Groundbreaking research reveals natural ways to boost ovulation and improve your chances of getting pregnant.* New York, NY: McGraw-Hill, 2008.

15. Gaskins AJ, Chiu YH, Williams PL, et al. Maternal whole grain intake and outcomes of in vitro fertilization. *Fertil Steril.* 2016; S0015-0282(16)00099-6. doi: 10.1016/j.fertnstert.2016.02.015.

16. Pitchford P. *Healing with Whole Foods: Asian traditions and modern nutrition.* 3rd ed. Berkeley, CA: North Atlantic Books, 2002.

17. Choi JM, Lebwohl B, Wang J, Lee SK, et al. Increased prevalence of Celiac disease in patients with unexplained infertility in the United States: a prospective study. *J Reprod Med.* 2011;56(5-6):199–203.

18. The Huffington Post. My Milk Manifesto. http://www.huffingtonpost.com/david-katz-md/my-milk-manifesto_b_6786048.html. Updated March 2, 2015. Accessed July 30, 2016.

19. Sizer FS, Whitney E. *Nutrition Concepts and Controversies.* 13th ed. Belmont, CA: Cengage, 2014.

20. National Dairy Council. Resource Library. https://www.nationaldairycouncil.org/. Accessed July 22, 2016.

21. USDA Department of Agriculture Research Service. Branded Food Products Database. https://ndb.nal.usda.gov/ndb/foods/. Accessed July 22, 2016.

22. Greenlee AR, Arbuckle TE, and Chyou PH. Risk factors for female infertility in an agricultural region. *Epidemiology.* 2003; 14 (4): 429-426. doi: 10.1097/01.EDE.0000071407.15670.aaAfeiche

23. MC, Chiu YH, Gaskins AJ, et al. Dairy intake in relation to in vitro fertilization outcomes among women from a fertility clinic. *Hum Reprod.* 2016; 31(3): 563-71. doi: 10.1093/humrep/dev344.

24. Afeiche MC, Williams PL, Mendiola J, et al. Dairy food intake in relation to semen quality and reproductive hormone levels among physically active young men. *Hum Reprod.* 2013; 28 (8): 2265-75. doi:10.1093/humrep/det133.

25. Xia W, Chiu, YH, Afeiche MC, et al. Impact of men's dairy intake on assisted reproductive technology outcomes among couples attending a fertility clinic. *Andrology.* 2016; 4: 277–283. doi:10.1111/andr.1215.

26. Chavarro JE, Rich-Edwards JW, Rosner BA, Willett WC. Diet and lifestyle in the prevention of ovulatory disorder infertility. *Obstet Gynecol.* 2007;110(5):1050–1058. doi:10.1097/01.AOG.0000287293.25465.

27. Vanegas JC, Afeiche MC, Gaskins AJ, et al. Soy food intake and treatment outcomes of women undergoing assisted reproductive technology. HHS Public Access. *Proc SPIE—the Int Soc Opt Eng*. 2015;73(4):389–400. doi:10.1530/ERC-14-0411.

28. Esmaeili V, Shahverdi a H, Moghadasian MH, Alizadeh a R. Dietary fatty acids affect semen quality: a review. *Andrology*. 2015:1–12. doi:10.1111/andr.12024.

29. Chavarro JE, Mínguez-Alarcón L, Mendiola J, Cutillas-Tolín A, López-Espín JJ, Torres-Cantero AM. Trans fatty acid intake is inversely related to total sperm count in young healthy men. *Hum Reprod*. 2014;29(3):429–40. doi:10.1093/humrep/det464.

30. Hammiche F, Vujkovic M, Wijburg W, et al. Increased preconception omega-3 polyunsaturated fatty acid intake improves embryo morphology. *Fertil Steril*. 2011;95(5):1820–1823. doi:10.1016/j.fertnstert.2010.11.021.

31. Jungheim ES, Frolova AI, Jiang H, Riley JK. Relationship between serum polyunsaturated fatty acids and pregnancy in women undergoing in vitro fertilization. *J Clin Endocrinol Metab*. 2013;98(8):E1364–8. doi:10.1210/jc.2012-4115.

32. Wathes DC, Abayasekara DRE, Aitken RJ. Polyunsaturated fatty acids in male and female reproduction. *Biol Reprod*. 2007;77(2):190–201. doi:10.1095/biolreprod.107.060558.

33. Health.gov. Scientific Report of the 2015 Dietary Guidelines Advisory Committee. https://health.gov/dietaryguidelines/2015-scientific-report/06-chapter-1/d1-2.asp. Updated September 2016. Accessed July 30, 2016.

34. Moslemi M, Tavanbakhsh S. Selenium–vitamin E supplementation in infertile men: effects on semen parameters and pregnancy rate. *Int J Gen Med*. 2011; 4: 99–104. doi: 10.2147/IJGM.S16275.

35. Endocrine Society. Vitamin D Deficiency May Reduce Pregnancy Rate in Women Undergoing IVF. https://www.endocrine.org/news-room/press-release-archives/2014/vitamin-d-deficiency-may-reduce-pregnancy-rate-in-women-undergoing-ivf. Accessed on August 1, 2016.

36. Food and Drug Administration. Food Safety at Home. http://www.fda.gov/forconsumers/byaudience/forwomen/ucm118524.htm. Updated on May 27, 2016. Accessed on July 30, 2016.

37. Academy of Nutrition and Dietetics. Storage in the Fridge. http://www.eatright.org/resource/homefoodsafety/four-steps/refrigerate/storage-in-the-fridge. Updated June 23, 2015. Accessed on August 3, 2016.

38. USDA Dietary Reference Intakes. DRI Nutrient Reports. https://fnic.nal.usda.gov/dietary-guidance/dietary-reference-intakes. Updated 2005. Accessed on July 1, 2016.

39. Whole Grain Council. Whole Grain Stamp. http://wholegrainscouncil.org/whole-grain-stamp. Accessed July 10, 2016.

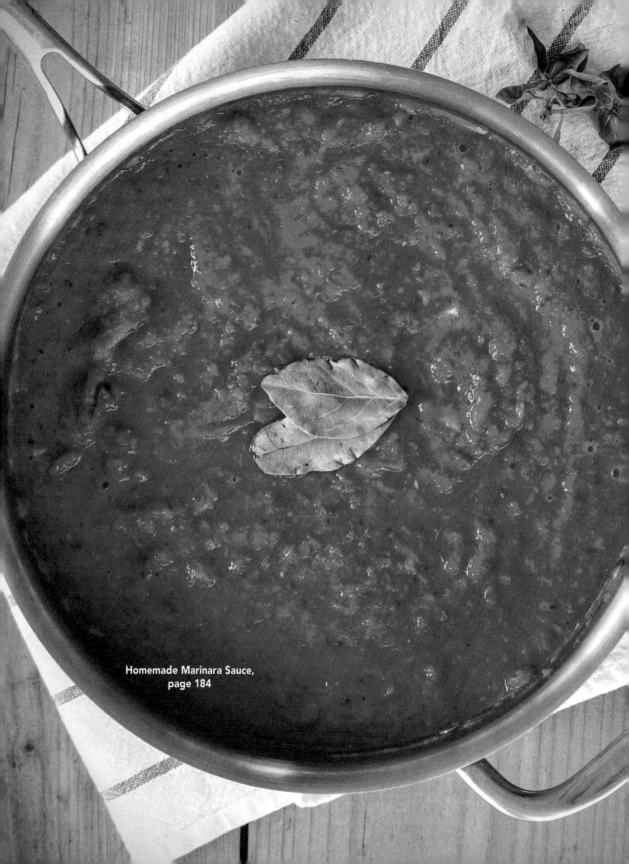

Homemade Marinara Sauce,
page 184

ABOUT THE AUTHORS

ELIZABETH SHAW, MS, RDN, CLT

Elizabeth Shaw has been a registered dietitian nutritionist for over six years. The unique positions she has held in the field of nutrition have helped her see the power nutrition has in public education.

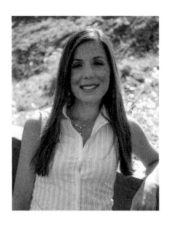

Elizabeth is a nutrition expert and serves as a nutrition communications and product development specialist. A guest on regional television, she hosts healthy living segments that highlight the ease of incorporating nutrient-dense recipes into meal planning. In addition, she is a freelance writer and serves as a nutrition expert for many national publications, such as the *Academy of Nutrition and Dietetics Food and Nutrition Magazine, Stone Soup Blog, Shape.com, Womens Health, Mens Health, Mens Fitness, Self, Reader's Digest, FitPregnancy.com, Today's Dietitian, FitnessMagazine.com, Parents.com* and others.

Elizabeth believes all foods can fit in a balanced lifestyle. She shares her passion for cooking and life on her blog, Shaw's Simple Swaps, and in her work as a professor in the San Diego Community College system where she teaches Introductory Nutrition, Advanced Nutrition and Cultural Foods as an online instructor.

Elizabeth also runs a website, www.BumpstoBaby.com, in which she shares her personal struggles with fertility. In this she provides comfort, support and health coaching for clients looking to work with a Registered Dietitian Nutritionist to help nurture their diet while struggling with infertility.

Elizabeth received her Master's in Nutrition as part of dual program during her Dietetic Internship at Northern Illinois University outside Chicago. She also completed a Graduate Program in Eating Disorders and Obesity there as well. She is a CLT (certified lifestyle eating and performance therapist) and uses that skillset to assist those with food allergies and intolerances. She holds a leadership role within the Nutrition Entrepreneurs Practice Group as Mentorship Chair.

CHEF SARA HAAS, RDN, LDN

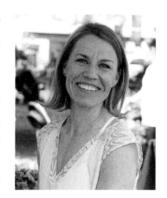

A food and nutrition expert with formal training in culinary arts, Sara has been a registered and licensed dietitian since 2002 and a professional chef since 2008. Working as a freelance writer, recipe developer, media authority, and consultant dietitian/chef, her clients include The Academy of Nutrition and Dietetics, *Eating Well Magazine, Shape Magazine,* Luvo, Leo Burnett Advertising Agency, *Parents.com, Food and Nutrition Magazine, Stack.com* and *Plan to Eat.*

She is a past National Academy of Nutrition and Dietetics Media Spokesperson, lending her talents to all forms of media, and has been featured in *Shape Magazine, U.S.A. Today, The Wall Street Journal, The Huffington Post, Epicurious.com, BabyCenter.com, O Magazine* and *Today's Dietitian Magazine.*

Sara is a contributing writer for *Eating Well Magazine as well as Food and Nutrition Magazine* and writes for its *Stone Soup* blog. She is a feed editor for The Feed Feed and has created recipes for organizations including Kids Eat Right and the Hass Avocado Board. In addition, Sara is the voice of the "Eating Right" minute, publicizing key nutrition messages on WBBM Newsradio 780 AM and 105.9 FM. Sara also shares her love of food and nutrition on her website, www.sarahaasrdn, where she posts recipes and nutrition related blog posts.

Sara graduated from Indiana University with a Bachelor of Science degree in Nutrition and Dietetics, completed her dietetic internship at the University of Massachusetts and earned her associates degree in culinary arts at The Cooking and Hospitality Institute of Chicago, Le Cordon Bleu Program. She is a member of the Academy of Nutrition and Dietetics, the Chicago Academy of Nutrition and Dietetics, the Food and Culinary Professionals Dietetic Practice Group and she is also a member of the Nutrition Entrepreneurs Dietetic Practice Group where she serves on the Executive Committee as Incoming Director of Awards and Networking.

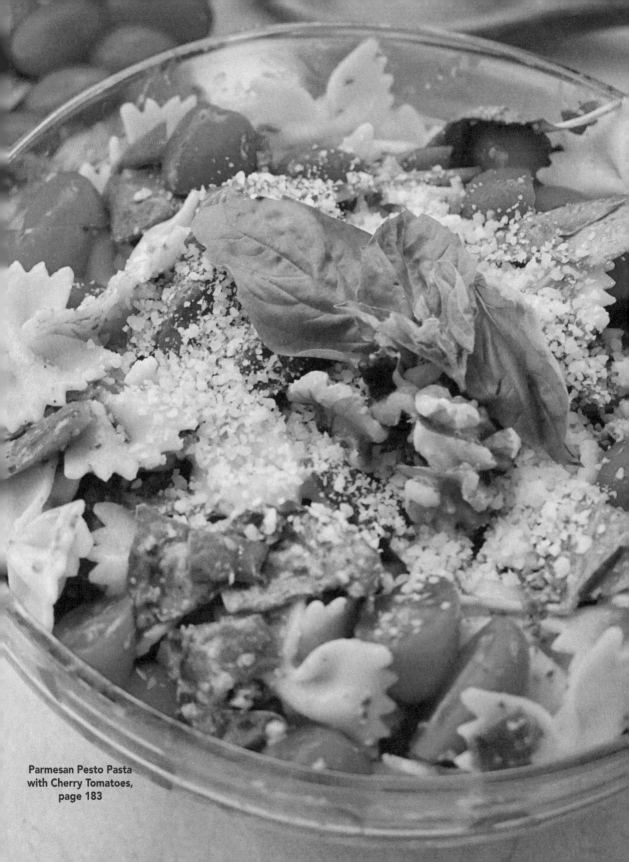

Parmesan Pesto Pasta
with Cherry Tomatoes,
page 183

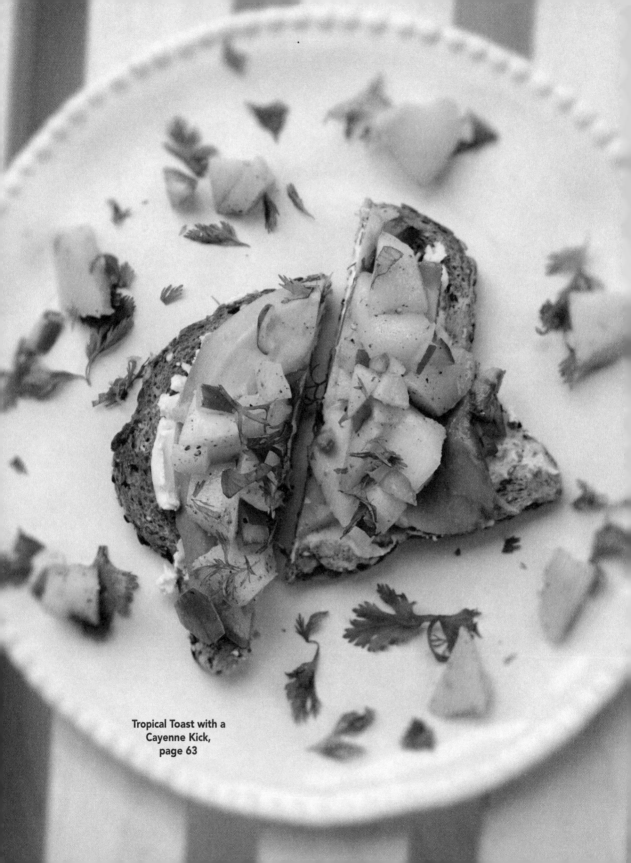

Tropical Toast with a Cayenne Kick, page 63

RECIPE INDEX

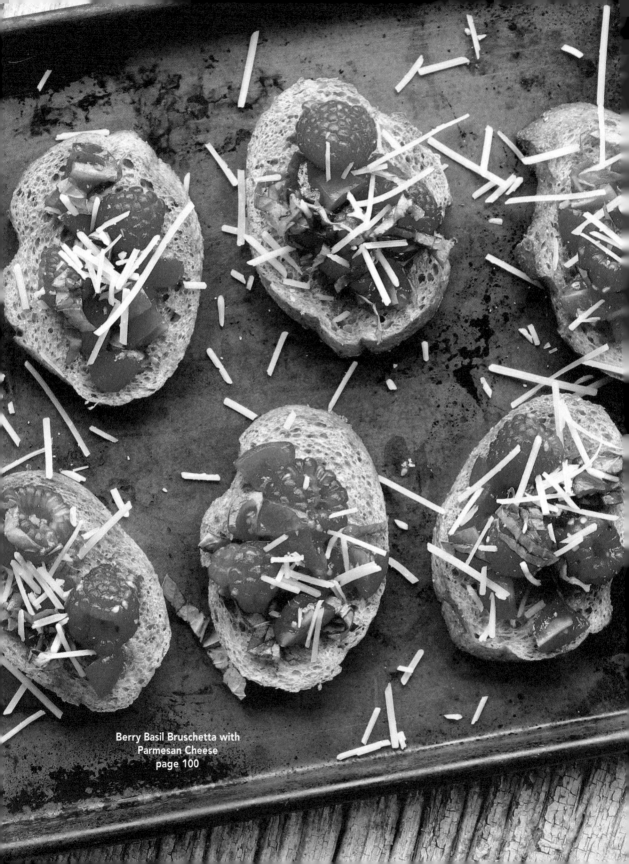

Berry Basil Bruschetta with
Parmesan Cheese
page 100

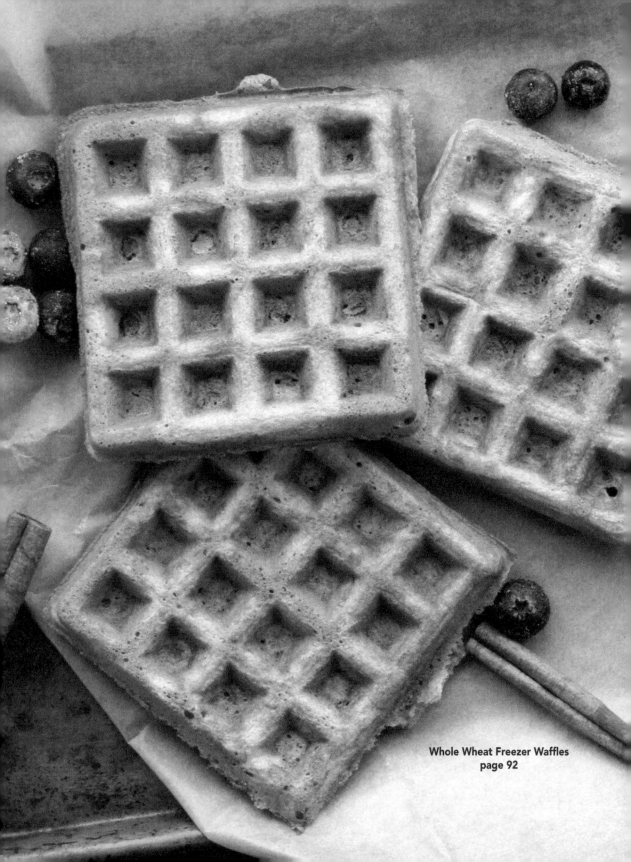

Whole Wheat Freezer Waffles
page 92

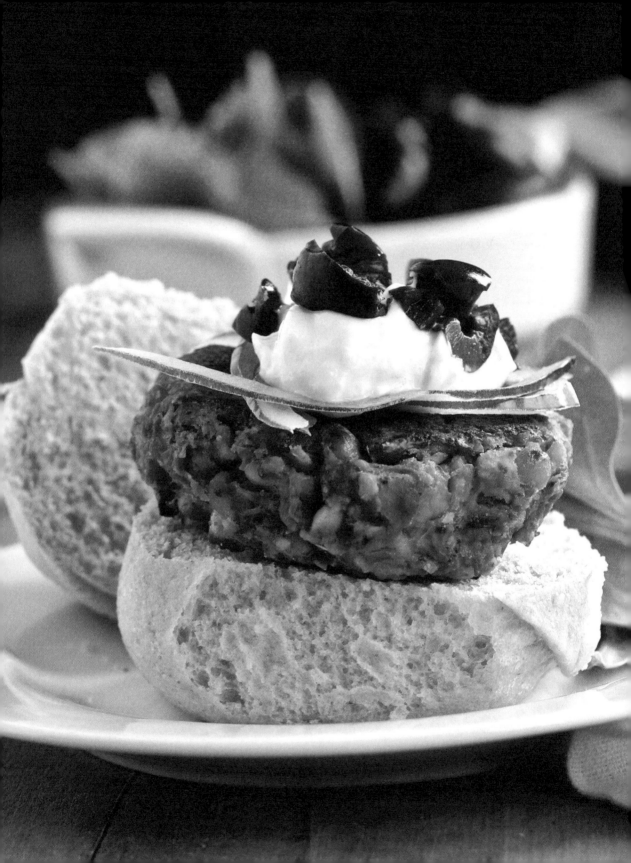

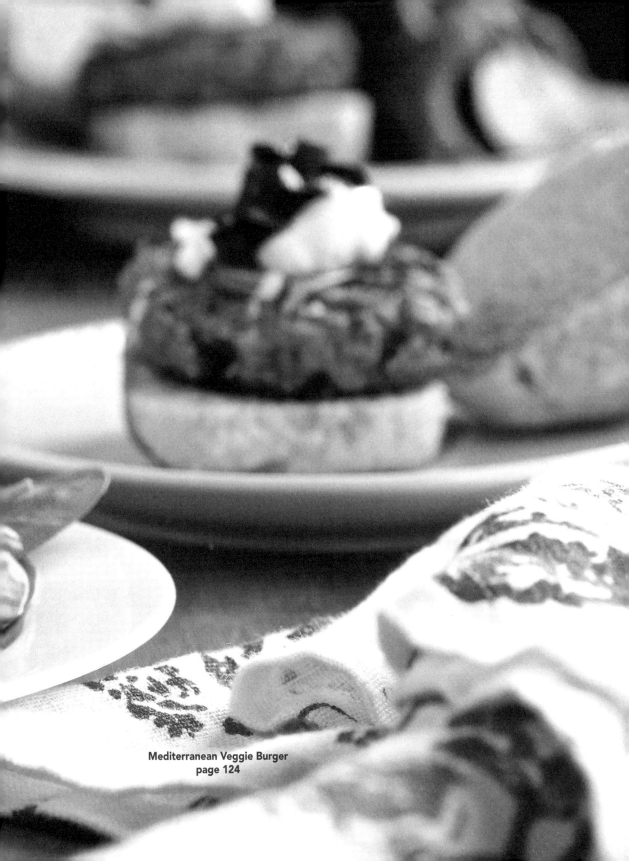

Mediterranean Veggie Burger
page 124